PEDIATRICS, CHILD AND ADOLESCENT HEALTH

SOFT SKILLS AND ASPIRATIONS IN CHINESE CHILDREN AND YOUTH

PEDIATRICS, CHILD AND ADOLESCENT HEALTH

JOAV MERRICK - SERIES EDITOR

NATIONAL INSTITUTE OF CHILD HEALTH AND HUMAN DEVELOPMENT,
MINISTRY OF SOCIAL AFFAIRS, JERUSALEM

Soft Skills and Aspirations in Chinese Children and Youth
Daniel TL Shek, Janet TY Leung, and Joav Merrick (Editors)
2018. ISBN: 978-1-53614-092-7 (Hardcover)
2018. ISBN: 978-1-53614-093-4 (e-book)

Building Youth for the Future: A Path towards Suicide Prevention
Hatim A Omar and Joav Merrick (Editors)
2018. ISBN: 978-1-53613-768-2 (Hardcover)
2018. ISBN: 978-1-53613-769-9 (e-book)

Child Health and Human Development Yearbook 2017
Joav Merrick (Editor)
2018. ISBN: 978-1-53613-628-9 (Hardcover)
2018. ISBN: 978-1-53613-629-6 (e-book)

Child and Adolescent Health Yearbook 2017
Joav Merrick (Editor)
2018. ISBN: 978-1-53613-594-7 (Hardcover)
2018. ISBN: 978-1-53613-595-4 (e-book)

Chronic Disease and Disability: The Pediatric Gastrointestinal Tract
Donald E Greydanus, Orhan Atay, and Joav Merrick (Editors)
2018. ISBN: 978-1-53612-948-9 (Hardcover)
2018. ISBN: 978-1-53612-949-6 (e-book)

Multiple Sclerosis in Children and Adolescents
Hatim Omar and Joshua Chalkley (Editors)
2018. ISBN: 978-1-53612-979-3 (Hardcover)
2018. ISBN: 978-1-53612-980-9 (e-book)

Childhood and Adolescence: Tribute to Emanuel Chigier, 1928-2017
Joav Merrick (Editor)
2018. ISBN: 978-1-53613-574-9 (Softcover)
2018. ISBN: 978-1-53613-575-6 (e book)

Chronic Disease and Disability: The Pediatric Lung
Donald E Greydanus, Myrtha M Gregoire-Bottex, Kevin W Cates and Joav Merrick (Editors)
2018. ISBN: 978-1-53613-577-0 (Hardcover)
2018. ISBN: 978-1-53613-578-7 (e-book)

Bicycles: Helmet Use of Adolescents at Independent Schools
Ronald Chow, Michael Borean, Drew Hollenberg, Jaclyn Viehweger, Tharani Anpalagan and Anna Rzepka (Editors)
2017. ISBN: 978-1-53612-458-3 (Hardcover)
2017. ISBN: 978-1-53612-459-0 (e-book)

Positive Youth Development: Long Term Effects in a Chinese Program
Daniel TL Shek, Cecilia MS Ma, Janet TY Leung and Joav Merrick (Editors)
2017. ISBN: 978-1-53612-539-9 (Hardcover)
2017. ISBN: 978-1-53612-540-5 (e-book)

Adolescence: Bicycle and Helmet Use of Adolescents and Young Adults
Ronald Chow and Joav Merrick (Editors)
2017. ISBN: 978-1-53612-039-4 (Hardcover)
2017. ISBN: 978-1-53612-060-8 (e-book)

Suicide: A Global View on Suicidal Ideation among Adolescents
Mazyanga L. Mazaba, Seter Siziya and Joav Merrick (Editors)
2017. ISBN: 978-1-53611-788-2 (Hardcover)
2017. ISBN: 978-1-53611-799-8 (e-book)

Children and Youth: Post-Traumatic Stress Disorder and Motor Vehicle Crashes
Donald E. Greydanus, Roger W. Apple, Kathryn White, and Joav Merrick (Editors)
2017. ISBN: 978-1-53611-102-6 (Hardcover)
2017. ISBN: 978-1-53611-255-9 (e-book)

Child and Adolescent Health Yearbook 2016
Joav Merrick (Editor)
2017. ISBN: 978-1-53610-948-1 (Hardcover)
2017. ISBN: 978-1-53610-957-3 (e-book)

Child Health and Human Development Yearbook 2016
Joav Merrick (Editor)
2017. ISBN: 978-1-53610-946-7 (Hardcover)
2017. ISBN: 978-1-53610-958-0 (e-book)

Chronic Disease and Disability: The Pediatric Kidney
Donald E Greydanus, Vimal Master Sankar Raj, and Joav Merrick (Editors)
2016. ISBN: 978-1-63483-793-4 (Hardcover)
2015. ISBN: 978-1-63483-809-2 (e-book)

Child and Adolescent Health Yearbook 2015
Joav Merrick (Editor)
2016. ISBN: 978-1-63484-512-0 (Hardcover)
2016. ISBN: 978-1-63484-543-4 (e-book)

Child Health and Human Development Yearbook 2015
Joav Merrick (Editor)
2016. ISBN: 978-1-63484-513-7 (Hardcover)
2016. ISBN: 978-1-63484-544-1 (e-book)

Pain Management Yearbook 2015
Joav Merrick (Editor)
2016. ISBN: 978-1-63484-515-1 (Hardcover)
2016. ISBN: 978-1-63484-545-8 (e-book)

Children and Childhood: Some International Aspects
Joav Merrick (Editor)
2016. ISBN: 978-1-63484-587-8 (Hardcover)
2016. ISBN: 978-1-63484-594-6 (e-book)

Children and Adolescents: Future Challenges
Daniel TL Shek, Tak Yan Lee, and Joav Merrick (Editors)
2016. ISBN: 978-1-63484-616-5 (Hardcover)
2016. ISBN: 978-1-63484-627-1 (e-book)

Adolescence: Positive Youth Development Programs in Chinese Communities
Daniel TL Shek, Florence KY Wu, Janet TY Leung, and Joav Merrick (Editors)
2016. ISBN: 978-1-63484-044-6 (Hardcover)
2016. ISBN: 978-1-63484-677-6 (e-book)

Sexuality: Some International Aspects
Joav Merrick and Donald E Greydanus (Editors)
2016. ISBN: 978-1-63484-707-0 (Hardcover)
2016. ISBN: 978-1-63484-719-3 (e book)

Growing Up in the Middle East: The Daily Lives and Well-Being of Israeli and Palestinian Youth
Yossi Harel-Fisch, Ziad Abdeen and Miriam Navot
2016. ISBN: 978-1-63484-746-9 (Hardcover)
2016. ISBN: 978-1-63484-765-0 (e-book)

Chronic Disease and Disability: The Pediatric Heart
Donald E Greydanus, Devika Malhotra and Joav Merrick (Editors)
2016. ISBN: 978-1-63484-828-2 (Hardcover)
2016. ISBN: 978-1-63484-842-8 (e-book)

Diabetes Mellitus: Childhood and Adolescence
Manmohan K Kamboj, Donald E Greydanus and Joav Merrick (Editors)
2016. ISBN: 978-1-53610-095-2 (Hardcover)
2016. ISBN: 978-1-53610-104-1 (e-book)

Chronic Disease and Disability: Abuse and Neglect in Childhood and Adolescence
Donald E Greydanus, Vincent J Palusci and Joav Merrick (Editors)
2016. ISBN: 978-1-53610-129-4 (Hardcover)
2016. ISBN: 978-1-53610-142-3 (e-book)

Clinical Aspects of Psychopharmacology in Childhood and Adolescence, Second Edition
Donald E Greydanus, Joseph L Calles, Jr, Dilip R Patel, Ahsan Nazeer and Joav Merrick (Editors)
2016. ISBN: 978-1-53610-241-3 (Hardcover)
2016. ISBN: 978-1-53610-253-6 (e-book)

Chronic Disease and Disability: The Pediatric Pancreas
Donald E Greydanus, Manmohan K Kamboj and Joav Merrick (Editors)
2016. ISBN: 978-1-53610-055-6 (Hardcover)
2016. ISBN: 978-1-53610-065-5 (e-book)

A Pediatric Resident Pocket Guide: Making the Most of Morning Reports
Arthur N Feinberg
2015. ISBN: 978-1-63482-141-4 (Softcover)
2015. ISBN: 978-1-63482-186-5 (e-book)

Tropical Pediatrics: A Public Health Concern of International Proportions Second Edition
Richard R Roach, Donald E Greydanus, Dilip R Patel and Joav Merrick (Editors)
2015. ISBN: 978-1-63463-381-9 (Hardcover)
2015. ISBN: 978-1-63463-404-5 (e-book)

Child and Adolescent Health Issues (A Tribute to the Pediatrician Donald E Greydanus)
Joav Merrick (Editor)
2015. ISBN: 978-1-63463-574-5 (Hardcover)
2015. ISBN: 978-1-63463-576-9 (e-book)

Child and Adolescent Health Yearbook 2014
Joav Merrick (Editor)
2015. ISBN: 978-1-63482-162-9 (Hardcover)
2015. ISBN: 978-1-63482-206-0 (e-book)

Child Health and Human Development Yearbook 2014
Joav Merrick (Editor)
2015. ISBN: 978-1-63482-163-6 (Hardcover)
2015. ISBN: 978-1-63482-207-7 (e-book)

Behavioral Pediatrics, 4th Edition
Donald E Greydanus, Dilip R Patel, Helen D Pratt, Joseph L Calles Jr, Ahsan Nazeer and Joav Merrick (Editors)
2015. ISBN: 978-1-63483-027-0 (Hardcover)
2015. ISBN: 978-1-63483-052-2 (e-book)

Disability, Chronic Disease and Human Development
Joav Merrick
2015. ISBN: 978-1-63483-029-4 (Hardcover)
2015. ISBN: 978-1-63483-057-7 (e-book)

Caribbean Adolescents: Some Public Health Concerns
Cecilia Hegamin-Younge and Joav Merrick (Editors)
2015. ISBN: 978-1-63483-341-7 (Hardcover)
2015. ISBN: 978-1-63483-343-1 (e-book)

Adolescence and Health: Some International Perspectives
Joav Merrick (Editor)
2015. ISBN: 978-1-63483-791-0 (Hardcover)
2015. ISBN: 978-1-63483-808-5 (e-book)

Youth Suicide Prevention: Everybody's Business
Hatim A Omar (Editor)
2015. ISBN: 978-1-63483-786-6 (Softcover)
2015. ISBN: 978-1-63483-820-7 (e-book)

Human Developmental Research: Experience from Research in Hong Kong
Daniel TL Shek, Cecilia Ma, Yu Lu and Joav Merrick (Editors)
2014. ISBN: 978-1-62808-166-4 (Hardcover)
2013. ISBN: 978-1-62808-167-1 (e-book)

School, Adolescence and Health Issues
Joav Merrick, Ariel Tenenbaum and Hatim A Omar (Editors)
2014. ISBN: 978-1-62948-702-1 (Hardcover)
2014. ISBN: 978-1-62948-707-6 (e-book)

Adolescence and Sexuality: International Perspectives
Joav Merrick, Ariel Tenenbaum and Hatim A Omar (Editors)
2014. ISBN: 978-1-62948-711-3 (Hardcover)
2014. ISBN: 978-1-62948-724-3 (e-book)

Child and Adolescent Health Yearbook 2013
Joav Merrick (Editor)
2014. ISBN: 978-1-63117-658-6 (Hardcover)
2014. ISBN: 978-1-63117-668-5 (e-book)

Adoption: The Search for a New Parenthood
Gary Diamond and Eva Arbel (Israel)
2014. ISBN: 978-1-63117-710-1 (Hardcover)
2014. ISBN: 978-1-63117-713-2 (e-book)

Adolescence: Places and Spaces
Myra F Taylor, Julie Ann Pooley and Joav Merrick (Editors)
2014. ISBN: 978-1-63117-847-4 (Hardcover)
2014. ISBN: 978-1-63117-850-4 (e-book)

Pain Management Yearbook 2013
Joav Merrick (Editor)
2014. ISBN: 978-1-63117-944-0 (Hardcover)
2014. ISBN: 978-1-63117-959-4 (e-book)

Child Health and Human Development Yearbook 2013
Joav Merrick (Editor)
2014. ISBN: 978-1-63117-939-6 (Hardcover)
2013. ISBN: 978-1-63117-958-7 (e-book)

Born into this World: Health Issues
Donald E Greydanus, Arthur N Feinberg, and Joav Merrick (Editors)
2014. ISBN: 978-1-63321-667-9 (Hardcover)
2014. ISBN: 978-1-63321-669-3 (e-book)

Caring for the Newborn: A Comprehensive Guide for the Clinician
Donald E Greydanus, Arthur N Feinberg and Joav Merrick (Editors)
2014. ISBN: 978-1-63321-760-7 (Hardcover)
2014. ISBN: 978-1-63321-781-2 (e-book)

Environment and Hope: Improving Health, Reducing AIDS and Promoting Food Security in the World
Leslie Rubin and Joav Merrick (Editors)
2014. ISBN: 978-1-63321-772-0 (Hardcover)
2014. ISBN: 978-1-63321-782-9 (e-book)

Pediatric and Adolescent Dermatology: Some Current Issues
Donald E Greydanus, Arthur N Feinberg and Joav Merrick (Editors)
2014. ISBN: 978-1-63321-853-6 (Hardcover)
2014. ISBN: 978-1-63321-863-5 (e-book)

Adolescence and Behavior Issues in a Chinese Context
Daniel TL Shek, Rachel CF Sun, and Joav Merrick (Editors)
2013. ISBN: 978-1-62618-614-9 (Hardcover)
2013. ISBN: 978-1-62618-692-7 (e-book)

Advances in Preterm Infant Research
Jing Sun, Nicholas Buys and Joav Merrick (Editors)
2013. ISBN: 978-1-62618-696-5 (Hardcover)
2013. ISBN: 978-1-62618-775-7 (e-book)

Child Health and Human Development: Social, Economic and Environmental Factors
Leslie Rubin and Joav Merrick (Editors)
2013. ISBN: 978-1-62948-166-1 (Hardcover)
2013. ISBN: 978-1-62948-169-2 (e-book)

Children, Violence and Bullying: International Perspectives
Joav Merrick, Isack Kandel and Hatim A Omar (Editors)
2013. ISBN: 978-1-62948-342-9 (Hardcover)
2013. ISBN: 978-1-62948-345-0 (e-book)

Chinese Adolescent Development: Economic Disadvantages, Parents and Intrapersonal Development
Daniel TL Shek, Rachel CF Sun and Joav Merrick (Editors)
2013. ISBN: 978-1-62618-622-4 (Hardcover)
2013. ISBN: 978-1-62618-694-1 (e-book)

Chronic Disease and Disability in Childhood
Joav Merrick (Editor)
2013. ISBN: 978-1-62808-865-6 (Hardcover)
2013. ISBN: 978-1-62808-868-7 (e-book)

Environmental Health Disparities in Children: Asthma, Obesity and Food
Leslie Rubin and Joav Merrick (Editors)
2013. ISBN: 978-1-62948-122-7 (Hardcover)
2013. ISBN: 978-1-62948-135-7 (e-book)

Environmental Health: Home, School and Community
Leslie Rubin and Joav Merrick (Editors)
2013. ISBN: 978-1-62948-155-5 (Hardcover)
2013. ISBN: 978-1-62948-158-6 (e-book)

Guidelines for the Healthy Integration of the Ill Child in the Educational System: Experience from Israel
Yosefa Isenberg
2013. ISBN: 978-1-62808-350-7 (Hardcover)
2013. ISBN: 978-1-62808-353-8 (e-book)

Internet Addiction: A Public Health Concern in Adolescence
Artemis Tsitsika, Mari Janikian, Donald E Greydanus, Hatim A Omar and Joav Merrick (Editors)
2013. ISBN: 978-1-62618-925-6 (Hardcover)
2013. ISBN: 978-1-62618-959-1 (e-book)

Playing with Fire: Children, Adolescents and Firesetting
Hatim A. Omar, Carrie Howell Bowling and Joav Merrick (Editors)
2013. ISBN: 978-1-62948-471-6 (Softcover)
2013. ISBN: 978-1-62948-474-7 (e-book)

Promotion of Holistic Development of Young People in Hong Kong
Daniel TL Shek, Tak Yan Lee and Joav Merrick (Editors)
2013. ISBN: 978-1-62808-019-3 (Hardcover)
2013. ISBN: 978-1-62808-040-7 (e-book)

University and College Students: Health and Development Issues for the Leaders of Tomorrow
Daniel TL Shek, Rachel CF Sun and Joav Merrick (Editors)
2013. ISBN: 978-1-62618-586-9 (Hardcover)
2013. ISBN: 978-1-62618-612-5 (e-book)

Break the Cycle of Environmental Health Disparities: Maternal and Child Health Aspects
Leslie Rubin and Joav Merrick (Editors)
2013. ISBN: 978-1-62948-107-4 (Hardcover)
2013. ISBN: 978-1-62948-133-3 (e-book)

Child and Adolescent Health Yearbook 2012
Joav Merrick (Editor)
2012. ISBN: 978-1-61942-788-4 (Hardcover)
2012. ISBN: 978-1-61942-789-1 (e-book)

Child Health and Human Development Yearbook 2011
Joav Merrick (Editor)
2012. ISBN: 978-1-61942-969-7 (Hardcover)
2012. ISBN: 978-1-61942-970-3 (e-book)

Child and Adolescent Health Yearbook 2011
Joav Merrick (Editor)
2012. ISBN: 978-1-61942-782-2 (Hardcover)
2012. ISBN: 978-1-61942-783-9 (e-book)

Tropical Pediatrics: A Public Health Concern of International Proportions
Richard R Roach, Donald E Greydanus, Dilip R Patel, Douglas N Homnick and Joav Merrick (Editors)
2012. ISBN: 978-1-61942-831-7 (Hardcover)
2012. ISBN: 978-1-61942-840-9 (e-book)

Child Health and Human Development Yearbook 2012
Joav Merrick (Editor)
2012. ISBN: 978-1-61942-978-9 (Hardcover)
2012. ISBN: 978-1-61942-979-6 (e-book)

Developmental Issues in Chinese Adolescents
Daniel TL Shek, Rachel CF Sun and Joav Merrick (Editors)
2012. ISBN: 978-1-62081-262-4 (Hardcover)
2012. ISBN: 978-1-62081-270-9 (e-book)

Positive Youth Development: Theory, Research and Application
Daniel TL Shek, Rachel CF Sun and Joav Merrick (Editors)
2012. ISBN: 978-1-62081-305-8 (Hardcover)
2012. ISBN: 978-1-62081-347-8 (e-book)

Understanding Autism Spectrum Disorder: Current Research Aspects
Ditza A Zachor and Joav Merrick (Editors)
2012. ISBN: 978-1-62081-353-9 (Hardcover)
2012. ISBN: 978-1-62081-390-4 (e-book)

Positive Youth Development: A New School Curriculum to Tackle Adolescent Developmental Issues
Hing Keung Ma, Daniel TL Shek and Joav Merrick (Editors)
2012. ISBN: 978-1-62081-384-3 (Hardcover)
2012. ISBN: 978-1-62081-385-0 (e-book)

Transition from Pediatric to Adult Medical Care
David Wood, John G Reiss, Maria E Ferris, Linda R Edwards and Joav Merrick (Editors)
2012. ISBN: 978-1-62081-409-3 (Hardcover)
2012. ISBN: 978-1-62081-412-3 (e-book)

PEDIATRICS, CHILD AND ADOLESCENT HEALTH

SOFT SKILLS AND ASPIRATIONS IN CHINESE CHILDREN AND YOUTH

DANIEL TL SHEK
JANET TY LEUNG
AND
JOAV MERRICK
EDITORS

nova
science publishers
New York

Additional color graphics may be available in the e-book version of this book.

Library of Congress Cataloging-in-Publication Data

ISBN: 978-1-53614-092-7

Published by Nova Science Publishers, Inc. Publishers, Inc. † New York

CONTENTS

INTRODUCTION

In: Soft Skills and Aspirations …
Editors: Daniel TL Shek, et al.
ISBN: 978-1-53614-092-7

Chapter 1

DEVELOPMENT OF "SOFT SKILLS" IN ADOLESCENTS

Daniel TL Shek[1-5,*], PhD, FHKPS, BBS, SBS, JP, Janet TY Leung[1], RSW, PhD and Joav Merrick[5-8], MD, MMedSci, DMSc

[1]Department of Applied Social Sciences,
The Hong Kong Polytechnic University, Hong Kong, PR China
[2]Centre for Innovative Programmes for Adolescents and Families,
The Hong Kong Polytechnic University, Hong Kong, PR China
[3]Department of Social Work, East China Normal University,
Shanghai, PR China
[4]Kiang Wu Nursing College of Macau, Macau, PR China
[5]Division of Adolescent Medicine, Kentucky Children's Hospital,
University of Kentucky, Lexington, Kentucky, US
[6]National Institute of Child Health and Human Development,
Jerusalem, Israel
[7]Department of Pediatrics, Hadassah-Hebrew University
Medical Center, Mount Scopus Campus, Jerusalem, Israel

[*] Corresponding Author Email: daniel.shek@polyu.edu.hk.

[8]Center for Healthy Development, School of Public Health, Georgia State University, Atlanta, US

Abstract

Young people are expected to learn "academic" or "technical" knowledge in a manufacturing economy, which can be referred to as "hard skills" such as to produce a television through the assembly lines. In many contemporary countries, we have observed a shift from manufacturing economy to service economy, which will result in young people expected to gain skills that are non-technical and widely transferable to different settings, termed "soft skills," which are basically related to the qualities of an individual. In this book, we include several chapters on soft skills development in adolescents with particular reference to the Chinese culture, including conclusions based on the data collected from the third year of the community-based P.A.T.H.S. Project in Hong Kong. We also discuss dreams, aspirations, hope and related constructs in Chinese adolescents. Besides, we also have chapters on the relationships between pornography consumption and positive youth development qualities. Finally, we document attempts to promote soft skills in university students. With the emergence and consolidation of service or knowledge-based economy, the desired qualities in adolescents have changed. Obviously, soft skills development plays an important role in the employability of young people. It is also vital to the whole-person development of young people.

Introduction

In the manufacturing economy, young people are expected to learn "academic" or "technical" knowledge, which enables them to contribute to industrial production. Generally speaking, the term "hard skills" is used to describe knowledge that is "prescribed" in one's formal qualification. An example of hard skills is how one can produce a car through the assembly lines. However, with a shift from manufacturing economy to service economy, young people are expected to gain skills that are non-technical and widely transferable to different settings, including work and non-work settings (1, 2). Such skills are often termed as "soft skills," which are basically related to the qualities of an individual (3). The term "soft skills" has been used interchangeably with other terms such as "generic skills," "skills of employability," or "people skills."

While some researchers regard "soft skills" as interpersonal skills or people skills that include communication, conflict resolution, and cross-cultural relationship skills, others have argued that "soft skills" go beyond interpersonal skills to include intrapersonal skills and personal qualities, such as personality, likeability and self-management skills, and virtues such as loyalty, honesty, integrity and resilience (4, 5). In short, soft skills include both intrapersonal and interpersonal relationship attributes.

IMPORTANCE OF SOFT SKILLS

Why are soft skills so important? Primarily, educators and researchers have linked this to employability. The basic argument is that with the change of the economy from manufacturing to service orientation, young people need to develop qualities beyond hard skills. For example, the National Association of Colleges and Employers in the United States (6) asked employers on the features they would look for in job application forms, the top six answers included leadership, teamwork ability, writing skills, ability to solve problems, occupational ethics, and numerical and logical skills. Based on the responses of around 2,200 employers from the United States, the findings revealed that that while 77% of employers regarded soft skills as important as hard skills, 16% of the respondents responded that soft skills are given higher importance than hard skills when they assessed the suitability of the job applicants (7).

Besides the instrumental reason of enhancing employability, soft skills play an important role in the holistic development of young people. In the past few decades, youth workers and theorists had pointed out that besides intellectual development, other aspects of youth development such as social-emotional learning (e.g., self-awareness, social awareness, interpersonal competence, responsible decision making and self-management) are equally important. Based on a review of 200 studies on programs attempting to promote soft skills in children and adolescents, Durlak and colleagues (8) showed that such programs were able to promote the holistic development of students, including their interpersonal, emotional, and academic developmental outcomes. In the area of positive youth development, research also showed that positive youth development attributes are important for the holistic development of adolescents (9). Unfortunately, evidence-based programs promoting soft skills development in young people are sparse (10). With reference to the university context, there is a neglect of training in soft skills for university students worldwide. The Higher Education Academy of the United Kingdom conducted a nationwide survey on student engagement based on more than 24,000 undergraduates (11). Results revealed that while undergraduates reported strong gains in "hard skills," they reported little improvements in "soft skills" such as citizenship, creativity, and development of personal values during their university years. In the United States, the Association of American Colleges and Universities also conducted a survey, which showed that only 25% of employers perceived that university graduates were well-prepared in critical thinking, analytical reasoning, effective communication, problem-solving, and innovation (12).

CHINESE CULTURE

In this book, we include several chapters on soft skills development in adolescents with particular reference to the Chinese culture. In the first four chapters, evaluation findings based on the data collected from the third year of the community-based P.A.T.H.S. Project in Hong Kong are reported. In the next three chapters, the findings based on a review study of dreams, aspirations, hope and related constructs in Chinese adolescents are presented. These chapters provide some pointers for nurturing dreams in Chinese adolescents. In the next three chapters, the relationships between pornography consumption and positive youth development qualities are explored. In the last two chapters, attempts to promote soft skills in university students are documented. In the first of the last two chapters, evaluation findings on a subject entitled "Service Leadership" are presented. In the final chapter, a study documenting the views of university students on the General University Requirements via a qualitative method is presented.

With the emergence and consolidation of service or knowledge-based economy, the desired qualities in adolescents have changed. Obviously, soft skills development plays an important role in the employability of young people. It is also vital to the whole-person development of young people.

ACKNOWLEDGMENTS

The chapters in this book are revised and adapted versions based on papers published in the *International Journal on Disability and Human Development* 2017;16 (4) issue with permission.

REFERENCES

[1] Shek DTL, Chung PPY, Leung H. Manufacturing economy vs. service economy: Implications for service leadership. Int J Diasbil Hum Dev 2015;14(3):205-15.

[2] Shek DTL, Chung PPY, Leung H. How unique is the service leadership model? A comparison with contemporary leadership approaches. Int J Disabil Hum Dev 2015;14(3):217-31.

[3] Bennett N, Dunne E, Carré C. Patterns of core and generic skills provision in higher education. Higher Educ 1999; 37(1):71-93.

[4] Robles MM. Executive perceptions of the top 10 soft skills needed in today's workplace. Bus Commun Q 2012; 75(4):453-65.

[5] Devadason ES, Subramaniam T, Daniel EGS. Final year undergraduates' perceptions of the integration of soft skills in the formal curriculum: A survey of Malaysian public universities. Asia Pac Educ Rev 2010; 11(3):321-48.

[6] National Association of Colleges and Employers (NACE). Job outlook: The candidate skills/qualities employers want, the influence of attributes. URL: http://www.naceweb.org/s11122014/job-outlook-skills-qualities-employers-want.aspx.

[7] CareerBuilder. Overwhelming majority of companies say soft skills are just as important as hard skills, according to a new CareerBuilder Survey. URL: http://www.careerbuilder.com/share/aboutus/pressreleasesdetail.aspx?sd=4/10/2014&id=pr817&ed=12/31/2014.

[8] Durlak JA, Weissberg RP, Dymnicki AB, Taylor RD, Schellinger KB. The impact of enhancing students' social and emotional learning: A meta-analysis of school-based universal interventions. Child Dev 2011;82(1):405-32.

[9] Shek DTL, Sun RCF. The Project P.A.T.H.S. in Hong Kong: Development, training, implementation, and evaluation. J Pediatr Adolesc Gynecol 2013;26(3):S2-9.

[10] Catalano RF, Fagan AA, Gavin LE, Greenberg MT, Irwin CE, Ross DA, Shek DTL. Worldwide application of prevention science in adolescent health. Lancet 2012;379(9826):1653-64.

[11] Buckley A. The UK Engagement Survey (UKES) 2015: Students' perceptions of skills development. URL: https://www.heacademy.ac.uk/sites/default/files/ukes_2015.pdf.

[12] Times Higher Education. US universities should follow UK in promoting students' soft skills. URL: https://www.timeshighereducation.com/comment/opinion/us-universities-should-follow-uk-in-promoting-students-soft-skills/2019081.article.

SECTION ONE: EVALUATION

In: Soft Skills and Aspirations …
Editors: Daniel TL Shek, et al.
ISBN: 978-1-53614-092-7

Chapter 2

PERCEIVED EFFECTIVENESS AND SATISFACTION OF A COMMUNITY-BASED POSITIVE YOUTH DEVELOPMENT PROGRAM

Daniel TL Shek[1-5,*], PhD, FHKPS, BBS, SBS, JP, Janet TY Leung[1], PhD and Kies SY Chan[1], BSSc, MSSc

[1]Department of Applied Social Sciences, The Hong Kong Polytechnic University, Hong Kong, PR China

[2]Centre for Innovative Programs for Adolescents and Families, The Hong Kong Polytechnic University, Hong Kong, PR China

[3]Department of Social Work, East China Normal University, Shanghai, PR China

[4]Kiang Wu Nursing College of Macau, Macau, PR China

[5]Division of Adolescent Medicine, Department of Pediatrics, Kentucky Children's Hospital, University of Kentucky School of Medicine, Lexington, Kentucky, US

---

[*] Corresponding Author Email: daniel.shek@polyu.edu.hk.

ABSTRACT

In this chapter, we examine participants' perceptions of a community-based positive youth development program (the Project P.A.T.H.S.) based on the responses of 16,420 junior secondary students who joined the program in 2015. Subjective outcome evaluation approach was adopted to examine the students' views of program content, program instructors, and program effectiveness. Consistent with previous studies, results showed that students generally perceived the program positively, and positive relationships were found amongst the three domains of evaluation. Multiple regression analyses showed that perceived program content and instructor qualities were significant predictors and could explain 35% of the variance in program effectiveness perceived by the participants. The present findings are basically consistent with previous subjective outcome evaluation findings derived from the school-based and community-based programs of the Project P.A.T.H.S. in Hong Kong.

INTRODUCTION

Youth problems such as violence, internet addiction, and substance abuse are widespread in many contemporary societies. Nowadays, youth problems are becoming more diverse, as well as highly shaped by the mass media and information spread through the Internet. For addressing "traditional" problem behaviors, such as substance abuse, school drop-out, smoking, and early sexual behaviors, many preventive programs have been developed in different countries using different intervention approaches such as psychoeducation and remedial intervention approach (1).

However, youth developmental problems vary across cultures and societies, and they change rapidly according to the value system and social context of each society. In Hong Kong, there are many emerging youth problems such as the increasing prevalence of Internet addiction, compensated dating, self-harm behavior, and cyberbullying, which have created challenges for policy makers, parents, teachers and youth workers in both prevention and remedial work.

Few validated adolescent prevention and development programs (2) have been conducted in Asian communities and these programs have mainly been prevention and single-domain programs such as programs for tackling substance abuse and mood disorders. In fact, most youth programs focusing on prevention of a single problem behavior or a single developmental issue are not ideal because adolescent developmental issues tend to co-exist (3). In addition, many studies have shown that reduction of risk factors (e.g., poverty, family conflict) and strengthening of protective factors (e.g., family support, self-esteem) could help adolescents adjust to developmental challenges and overcome developmental difficulties (3-5). Such work suggests that promotion of protective factors such as psychosocial competence and prosocial beliefs may help prevent not just one form of adolescent risk behavior that contributes to adolescent psychological well-being.

To promote holistic adolescent development, which would eventually lead to a reduction of adolescent risk behavior, The Hong Kong Jockey Club Charities Trust initiated a large-scale program named the Project P.A.T.H.S. (Positive Adolescent Training through Holistic Social Program) in collaboration with five universities in Hong Kong (3). The program utilized principles and concepts of the positive youth development (PYD) approach, which highlights the talents, interests, strengths, and potentials of adolescents rather than focuses on treatment and prevention of risky behaviors. In other words, the positive youth development approach actively promotes human development by considering the potential and capabilities of each individual human being. There are 15 positive youth development constructs underpinning the conceptual framework of P.A.T.H.S., which include self-determination, resilience, spirituality, and other personal capacities such as emotional competence and social competence. These constructs were identified by Catalano et al. (6) after reviewing more than 70 youth development programs in the United States.

The P.A.T.H.S. Project was initially launched in the 2005/06 academic year and the content was tailored for junior secondary students (i.e., Grade 7-9). The project was composed of two tiers – Tier 1 was targeted to promote holistic development for all Secondary 1 to 3 students, and Tier 2 program was designed for about one-fifth of junior secondary students who have greater psychological needs (7). The Tier 1 program was a universal curriculum-based program vital to positive youth development. Junior secondary students attended 10 to 20 hours of the program based on the PYD constructs. Besides, some developmental issues such as substance abuse, sexuality, and financial management were included in the program content. A training program for program instructors, who were mainly secondary school teachers and social workers, was provided to enable the instructors to better understand adolescent development, to prepare relevant knowledge, skills, attitude, and to establish mutual support networks amongst them. The effectiveness of the training program was also rigorously evaluated (8). Since its inception, the project has benefited more than 320 Hong Kong schools with a total of 284,400 students (as in December 2015). From 2013 to 2015, the project P.A.T.H.S. has been implemented by means of a community-based model. Compared to the school-based model adopted in the previous years, community approach was expected to promote collaborative participation amongst families, schools and community organizations, and to increase the diversity of student participants (9).

To understand the impact of the Project P.A.T.H.S., it is important to carry out program evaluation. Client satisfaction evaluation is a common approach widely used in many human service settings such as education, social work, and healthcare (10). Some researchers believe that client satisfaction serves as an important indicator of the quality and effectiveness of the program and it is an essential way to obtain feedbacks from clients or program participants for the improvement of service delivery (11). In this study, we investigated program effectiveness via the client satisfaction approach. Basically, we investigated whether the program participants were satisfied with the program content, instructor, and effectiveness. Besides, the inter-relationships amongst these three aspects of satisfaction and predictors of perceived program effectiveness were also studied.

Program evaluation is a process of examining whether a program is generating its desired outcomes or impacts. It is commonly used to indicate whether the program could achieve its goals and objectives, and to uncover the unintended effects of the program (11-12). Program outcome evaluation focuses on the effectiveness of intervention (e.g., teaching and learning activities) and the attainment of program goals. There are many factors affecting the effectiveness of a program. According to Chen (12), program evaluation should include considerations of program implementers (e.g., training, participant-implementer relationships), implementing organization (e.g., schools), service delivery methods (e.g., activity design), and target populations (e.g., students' characteristics). Educational research also suggest that school and classroom contexts, quality of instruction, group activities, teacher behaviors, and consistency of curriculum are factors affecting student learning in school contexts (13). Generally speaking, program effectiveness cannot be simply evaluated by one single facet of the program. Various aspects of the program should be examined simultaneously to get a comprehensive picture of program effectiveness.

Although the client satisfaction approach is widely adopted in program evaluation, it is argued that students' subjective feedbacks could not reflect the quality and effectiveness of the program. For example, Mark (14) argued that students in higher education tend to have more satisfaction when perceived performance meets their own expectations. The client satisfaction approach was also criticized because most of the studies reported that more than 75% of participants were satisfied with the program (15). These high satisfaction rates might be due to biases created by service providers such as using double questions and biased rating scales in the evaluation process (16). Besides, researchers (11) argued that participant satisfaction of various aspects of a program could not reflect whether the participants changed positively and the changes may not result from the program. Client satisfaction is also not a program outcome in general and participants are always satisfied if the implementation environment of the program could meet their own needs or preferences (17). Hence, the client satisfaction approach was said to be "not able to provide critical evidence of the effectiveness of the program" (18).

Despite the arguments against the value of the client satisfaction approach, program effectiveness evaluation and client satisfaction evaluation share common factors in explaining program outcomes. Elliott (19) found that "student centeredness" and "instructional effectiveness" are the major determinants of students' overall educational experience that influence student satisfaction, which suggests that institutional factors such as instructor's performance might affect client's satisfaction. Another study (20) on client satisfaction found that while both institutional (e.g., the student-teacher relationship) and social factors (e.g., social experience with other students) are significant predictors of client satisfaction, other factors such as student's personal background, learning environment and commitment to the school should also be considered. These findings are consistent with Chen's (12) study as abovementioned, which suggests that student characteristics, instructor quality, implementation process, and implementation environment are all predictors of program effectiveness.

Besides, other research findings also suggest that subjective outcome evaluation findings could predict program effectiveness to some degree. Shek (21) attempted to examine the relationship between subjective and objective outcome evaluation based on Chinese secondary students. Results showed that subjective outcome evaluation was highly correlated with objective outcome evaluation where the scores of subjective evaluations were positively associated with the changes in attitude and behavior reported by the program participants. Another study also showed a significant relationship between client satisfaction ratings and clients' progress of undergoing a child protection program, as well as between the client satisfaction level and their changes in child neglect behavior (22).

Despite the existence of different views on the value of the client satisfaction approach, client satisfaction ratings are commonly regarded as an important indicator of program success. Besides looking at the satisfaction levels of program participants, the present study also examined the inter-relationships between different aspects of client satisfaction and the determinants of perceived effectiveness. Regarding the latter, Shek and Sun (23) found that perceived program qualities and program implementers positively predicted program effectiveness ratings. Grade differences of subjective outcome evaluation ratings were also investigated in this study. Previous studies found that younger students always responded more positively as compared to higher grade students (23-25). These findings raised the question of whether there would be grade differences of subjective outcome evaluation in the current study.

In this study, the participants were junior secondary (Grade 7-9) students who had completed the Tier 1 program of the community-based P.A.T.H.S. Project. Several research questions were raised as follows:

1) How do the student participants evaluate the Tier 1 Program of the community-based P.A.T.H.S. Project? Based on the past findings (23-25) from different evaluation methods, it was expected that the participants would generally be satisfied with the program (Hypothesis 1).
2) What are the inter-relationships amongst the different aspects of client satisfaction, including perceived program quality, perceived instructor quality and perceived benefits of the program? Based on previous studies (23-25), it was predicted that these three aspects of client satisfaction would be significantly correlated amongst themselves (Hypotheses 2a, 2b and 2c).
3) Is there any difference in the subjective outcome evaluation ratings between the grades? From the previous findings (24-25), it was hypothesized that students in higher grades would be less satisfied than students in lower grades (Hypothesis 3).
4) Do perceived program quality and perceived instructor quality predict perceived program effectiveness? Based on previous studies (23-25), it was hypothesized that these two factors would predict perceived program effectiveness (Hypotheses 4a and 4b).

OUR STUDY

A total of 21 agencies had implemented the community-based program in 41 projects in community centers or schools located in different districts throughout Hong Kong. To implement the program, 358 social workers, and 254 teachers or teaching assistants were involved. In these projects, 18,384 secondary students participated in the program. Amongst them, 14,387 were Secondary 1 students (Grade 7), 2,373 were Secondary 2 students (Grade 8), and 1,624 were Secondary 3 students (Grade 9).

To facilitate the evaluation process, a briefing session was conducted with the agencies before the program implementation. After the Tier 1 Program was completed, all student participants were invited to fill in the Subjective Outcome Evaluation Form (Form A). During the administration, the principles of confidentiality, anonymity, voluntary participation and freedom to withdraw from the study were emphasized and consent was obtained from all participants. A total of 16,420 questionnaires were returned to the Research Team. Amongst them, 13,003 were Secondary 1 students, 1,989 were Secondary 2 students, and 1,415 were Secondary 3 students. The overall response rate was 89.32%.

Instruments

A validated instrument (Form A) was used to assess students' subjective evaluation of the program. It had four parts. Part 1 assessed participants' perceptions of the program content, such as program objectives, design, interaction among students, and level of participation (10 items). The second part assessed participants' perceptions of instructor's qualities, such as participation, attitude, and preparation of the instructors (10 items). Participants rated the items in the first two parts on a 6-point Likert scale, where 1 indicated *strongly disagree* and 6 indicated *strongly agree*. Part 3 assessed participants' perceptions of the program effectiveness (16 items). A 5-point Likert scale was employed with 1 indicating the program *unhelpful* and 6 indicating the program *really helpful*. The final Part consisted of three items, which measured the extent to which the participants would recommend the program to others, the extent to which the participants would participate in similar programs, and their overall satisfaction with the program. There were also four open-ended questions on participants' experiences with the program, such as things that they learned from the program and areas where the program should be improved. The open-ended part was not used for analysis in this study because of space limitation.

Data analyses

Reliability analysis was employed to test the internal consistency of the subjective outcome evaluation measures. Descriptive statistical analyses focusing on the percentage of responses to each item were carried out to reflect the participants' perceptions of the program qualities, instructor qualities, and program effectiveness (Hypothesis 1). For the relationships amongst various aspects of the evaluation measures, Pearson correlation analyses were carried out (Hypotheses 2a, 2b, & 2c). Regarding grade differences (Hypothesis 3), one-way ANOVAs were conducted to examine differences in the evaluation ratings amongst students in Secondary 1, 2 and 3 levels. Lastly, multiple regression analyses were conducted to examine whether program effectiveness could be predicted by program content or program instructors (Hypothesis 4). SPSS 22.0 was used for the present statistical analyses.

FINDINGS

Results on the internal consistency of Form A are shown in Table 1. It was found that the three parts in the questionnaire had high internal consistency. The alpha values were .97 for the 10 questions evaluating program content, .98 for the 10 questions evaluating program instructors, and .98 for the 16 questions evaluating program effectiveness. The Cronbach's alpha coefficient for the three parts of the evaluation (i.e., 36 items) was .98.

Results on the participants' evaluation of the program content are shown in Table 2. Most of the participants responded positively when evaluating the program content. For example, 89.7% felt that the activities in the curriculum were planned carefully; 89.0% agreed that the classroom atmosphere was very pleasant; 88.8% reported they experienced lots of peer interactions amongst students; and 87.9% agreed that they actively participated in the lessons. The item on the clarity of curriculum objectives got the highest rating of 89.8%. For the overall perception, 87.8% reported that on the whole, they liked the curriculum very much.

Table 3 shows the descriptive statistics on the evaluation of program instructors. Amongst the participants in all grade levels, all 10 items got more than 90% of positive ratings, including instructors' mastery of curriculum (91.2%), preparation for the lessons (91.7%), teaching skills (91.3%), and professional attitudes (91.6%). The participants also evaluated the instructors as very involved (91.9%), being able to encourage students' participation (91.7%), being caring toward the students (90.9%), and having lots of interactions with them (90.9%). The overall evaluation received the highest positive rating of 92.2%, reflecting the high satisfaction with the performance of program instructors.

Table 1. Mean, standard deviations, Cronbach's alphas, and mean inter-item correlations

	S1		S2		S3		Overall	
	M (SD)	α (Mean#)	M (SD)	α (Mean#)	M (SD)	α (Mean#)	M (SD)	α (Mean#)
Program content (10 items)	4.62 (.95)	.97 (.75)	4.58 (.90)	.97 (.74)	4.59 (.85)	.96 (.69)	4.62 (.94)	.97 (.75)
Program instructors (10 items)	4.80 (.95)	.98 (.81)	4.75 (.91)	.98 (.81)	4.77 (.86)	.97 (.76)	4.79 (.94)	.98 (.81)
Program effectiveness (16 items)	3.81 (.88)	.98 (.76)	3.61 (.85)	.98 (.76)	3.71 (.84)	.98 (.71)	3.78 (.86)	.98 (.75)
Total effectiveness (36 items)	4.30 (.79)	.98 (.58)	4.19 (.74)	.98 (.55)	4.22 (.73)	.98 (.53)	4.28 (.78)	.98 (.57)

Note: S1: Secondary 1 level; S2: Secondary 2 level; S3: Secondary 3 level.
Mean inter-item correlations.

Regarding the evaluation of program effectiveness, most participants perceived the program to be effective in fostering the specific qualities of positive youth development (Table 4).

Table 2. Descriptive statistics of the participants' evaluations on the program content

	Respondents with positive responses (Options 4-6)							
	S1		S2		S3		Overall	
	n	%	*n*	%	*n*	%	*N*	%
1. The objectives of the curriculum are very clear.	11606	89.9	1757	89.7	1253	89.4	14628	89.8
2. The design of the curriculum is very good.	11523	89.2	1756	89.5	1242	89.0	14532	89.2
3. The activities were carefully planned.	11584	89.7	1762	90.0	1249	89.3	14607	89.7
4. The classroom atmosphere was very pleasant.	11440	88.7	1762	90.0	1261	90.3	14475	89.0
5. There was a lot of peer interactions amongst the students.	11440	88.8	1730	88.7	1250	89.5	14432	88.8
6. I participated actively during lessons (including discussions, sharing, games, etc.).	11338	87.8	1700	86.8	1249	89.6	14298	87.9
7. I was encouraged to do my best.	11262	87.3	1654	84.4	1235	88.5	14162	87.1
8. The learning experience I encountered enhanced my interest towards the lessons.	11271	87.5	1685	86.1	1228	88.0	14194	87.3
9. Overall speaking, I have very positive evaluation of the program.	11342	87.9	1708	87.3	1249	89.5	14308	87.9
10. On the whole, I like this curriculum very much.	11314	87.8	1713	87.4	1242	89.0	14279	87.8

Note: All items are on a 6-point Likert scale with 1 = strongly disagree, 2 = disagree, 3 = slightly disagree, 4 = slightly agree, 5 = agree, 6 = strongly agree. Only respondents with positive responses (Options 4-6) are shown in the table. S1: Secondary 1 level; S2: Secondary 2 level; S3: Secondary 3 level.

For instance, the participants agreed that the program could strengthen their bonding with others (87.7%) and resilience (89.6%), improve their ability in emotional expression and management (89.9%), increase self-confidence (89.3%), and increase self-awareness (90.4%). The items receiving the highest ratings were "ability to distinguish between the good and the bad" (91.8%) and "increase competence in making sensible and wise choices" (91.7%). There were 91.7% of the participants agreeing that the program enriched their overall development.

Table 3. Descriptive statistics of the participants' evaluations of the program instructors

	Respondents with positive responses (Options 4-6)							
	S1		S2		S3		Overall	
	n	%	*n*	%	*n*	%	*N*	%
1. The instructor(s) had a good mastery of the curriculum.	11760	91.1	1793	91.3	1290	92.2	14852	91.2
2. The instructor(s) was well prepared for the lessons.	11833	91.6	1807	92.0	1287	92.1	14937	91.7
3. The instructor(s)' teaching skills were good.	11778	91.3	1794	91.5	1279	91.8	14861	91.3
4. The instructor(s) showed good professional attitudes.	11812	91.6	1802	91.9	1283	91.8	14907	91.6
5. The instructor(s) was very involved.	11841	91.8	1811	92.3	1297	93.0	14858	91.9
6. The instructor(s) encouraged students to participate in the activities.	11831	91.7	1800	91.6	1294	92.6	14934	91.7
7. The instructor(s) cared for the students.	11738	91.0	1776	90.4	1269	91.0	14792	90.9
8. The instructor(s) was ready to offer help to students when needed.	11861	91.9	1804	91.9	1279	91.8	14954	91.9
9. The instructor(s) had lots of interactions with the students.	11746	91.0	1781	90.7	1268	90.7	14803	90.9
10. Overall speaking, I have very positive evaluation of the instructors.	11890	92.1	1816	92.5	1302	93.1	15017	92.2

Note: All items are on a 6-point Likert scale with 1 = strongly disagree, 2 = disagree, 3 = slightly disagree, 4 = slightly agree, 5 = agree, 6 = strongly agree. Only respondents with positive responses (Options 4-6) are shown in the table. S1: Secondary 1 level; S2: Secondary 2 level; S3: Secondary 3 level.

Table 5 shows the participants' responses to the rest of the items in Form A. Specifically, 85.2% of the participants responded that they would suggest their friends to join the program, 76.1% said they were willing to participate in similar programs again in the future, and 95% indicated that they were satisfied with the program. These results suggest that participants generally viewed the program positively.

Table 4. Descriptive statistics of the participants' evaluations of the program effectiveness

The extent to which the course (i.e., the program that all students have joined) has helped you:	**Respondents with positive responses (Options 3-5)**							
	S1		S2		S3		Overall	
	n	%	*N*	%	*n*	%	*N*	%
1. It has strengthened my bonding with teachers, classmates and my family.	11084	88.0	1660	86.4	1184	86.9	13941	87.7
2. It has strengthened my resilience in adverse conditions.	11325	89.9	1712	88.9	1207	88.4	14257	89.6
3. It has enhanced my social competence.	11472	91.2	1732	89.7	1221	89.8	14438	90.9
4. It has improved my ability in handling and expressing my emotions.	11347	88.0	1701	88.6	1201	88.3	14262	89.9
5. It has enhanced my cognitive competence.	11412	90.7	1731	89.9	1214	89.1	14370	90.5
6. My ability to resist harmful influences has been improved.	11492	91.3	1742	90.7	1214	89.4	14461	91.1
7. It has strengthened my ability to distinguish between the good and the bad.	11594	92.1	1752	91.0	1225	90.1	14584	91.8
8. It has increased my competence in making sensible and wise choices.	11580	92.0	1747	90.8	1229	90.5	14569	91.7
9. It has helped me to have life reflections.	11313	90.0	1698	88.7	1208	89.3	14232	89.8
10. It has reinforced my self-confidence.	11289	89.7	1683	87.4	1204	88.5	14189	89.3
11. It has increased my self-awareness.	11413	90.7	1710	89.1	1211	89.0	14347	90.4
12. It has helped me to face the future with a positive attitude.	11432	90.9	1721	89.6	1232	90.6	14398	90.7
13. It has helped me to cultivate compassion and care about others.	11455	91.1	1714	89.1	1221	89.6	14403	90.7
14. It has encouraged me to care about the community.	11337	90.2	1700	88.8	1206	88.6	14256	89.9
15. It has promoted my sense of responsibility in serving the society.	11395	90.5	1691	88.3	1200	88.2	14299	90.0
16. It has enriched my overall development.	11568	91.9	1739	90.7	1239	91.0	14559	91.7

Note: All items are on a 5-point Likert scale with 1 = unhelpful, 2 = not very helpful, 3 = slightly helpful, 4 = helpful, 5 = very helpful. Only respondents with positive responses (Options 3-5) are shown in the table. S1: Secondary 1 level; S2: Secondary 2 level; S3: Secondary 3 level.

Table 5. Other aspects of subjective outcome evaluation based on the participants' perception

A. If your friends have needs and conditions similar to yours, will you suggest him/her to join this course?

Respondents with positive responses (Options 3-4)							
S1		S2		S3		Overall	
n	%	*n*	%	*n*	%	*N*	%
9943	85.1	1607	84.3	1143	87.9	12699	85.2

Note: The item is on a 4-point Likert scale with 1 = definitely will not suggest, 2 = will not suggest, 3 = will suggest, 4 = definitely will suggest. Only respondents with positive responses (Options 3-4) are shown in the table. S1: Secondary 1 level; S2: Secondary 2 level; S3: Secondary 3 level.

B. Will you participate in similar courses again in the future?

Respondents with positive responses (Options 3-4)							
S1		S2		S3		Overall	
n	%	*n*	%	*n*	%	*N*	%
8897	75.8	1441	75.1	1043	79.9	11385	76.1

Note: The item is on a 4-point Likert scale with 1 = definitely will not participate, 2 = will not participate, 3 = will participate, 4 = definitely will participate. Only respondents with positive responses (Options 3-4) are shown in the table. S1: Secondary 1 level; S2: Secondary 2 level; S3: Secondary 3 level.

C. On the whole, are you satisfied with this course?

Respondents with positive responses (Options 4-6)							
S1		S2		S3		Overall	
n	%	*n*	%	*n*	%	*N*	%
12166	94.78	1884	95.7	1334	95.8	15393	95.0

Note: All items are on a 6-point Likert scale with 1 = very dissatisfied, 2 = moderately dissatisfied, 3 = slightly dissatisfied, 4 = satisfied, 5 = moderately satisfied, 6 = very satisfied. Only respondents with positive responses (Options 4-6) are shown in the table. S1: Secondary 1 level; S2: Secondary 2 level; S3: Secondary 3 level.

To understand the relationships amongst the three aspects of subjective evaluation, Pearson correlation analyses were conducted (Table 6).

Results showed that the three aspects were significantly correlated amongst themselves. The relationship between perceived program content and perceived program instructor was the strongest (r = .79, p < .001). Perceived program effectiveness was also significantly related to program content (r = .58, p < .001) and program instructors (r = .51, p < .001).

Several One-way ANOVAs were conducted to analyze grade differences in the subjective outcome evaluation ratings, with grade level as the independent variable and perceived program content (10 items), instructors (10 items), program effectiveness (16 items), and total scale (36 items) as the dependent variables. Results in Table 7 showed that participants in different grades differed in their perception of program effectiveness (16 items) (F (2, 15,495) = 49.74, p < .001) and total program satisfaction (F (2, 15,047) = 19.29, p < .001). Post-hoc comparison tests with Bonferroni corrections further indicated that Secondary 1 students had significantly higher ratings on perceived program effectiveness and total program satisfaction compared to Secondary 2 and 3 participants. Secondary 2 students' ratings were also different from those of Secondary 3 students on the ratings of perceived program effectiveness.

Table 6. Pearson correlations amongst program content, instructors, and effectiveness

Variables	1	2	3
1. Program content (10 items)	-		
2. Program instructors (10 items)	.79**	-	
3. Program effectiveness (16 items)	.58**	.51**	-

** *p* < .001.

Multiple regression analyses were further employed to examine to what extent program content and program instructors predicted perceived program effectiveness (Table 8). Evaluation of program content was found to be a strong predictor for perceived program effectiveness among all the three grades (Secondary 1: β = .48, p < 0.001; Secondary 2: β = .40, p < 0.001; Secondary 3: β = .49, p < 0.001; overall: β = .47, p < 0.001).

Table 7. One-way ANOVA comparing the evaluations of the program of participants in different grade levels

		Sum of Squares	df	Mean Square	F
Program content	Between Groups	3.50	2	1.75	1.99
	Within Groups	14065.32	16011	.88	
	Total	14068.82	16013		
Program instructors	Between Groups	4.72	2	2.36	2.68
	Within Groups	14158.29	16097	.88	
	Total	14163.00	16099		
Program effectiveness	Between Groups	75.84	2	37.92	49.74**
	Within Groups	11812.37	15495	.76	
	Total	11888.21	15497		
Total effectiveness	Between Groups	23.30	2	11.65	19.29**
	Within Groups	9089.30	15047	.60	
	Total	9112.61	15049		

** $p < .001$.

Post Hoc Tests (Multiple comparisons)

Dependent Variables	(I) Grade	(J) Grade	Mean Difference (I-J)	Standard Error
Program content	S1	S2	.04	.02
		S3	.03	.03
	S2	S3	-.01	.03
Program instructors	S1	S2	.05	.02
		S3	.03	.03
	S2	S3	-.01	.03
Program effectiveness	S1	S2	.20**	.02
		S3	.11**	.03
	S2	S3	-.09*	.03
Total effectiveness	S1	S2	.11**	.02
		S3	.07*	.02
	S2	S3	-.04	.03

Note: S1: Secondary 1 level; S2: Secondary 2 level; S3: Secondary 3 level. * $p < .01$; ** $p < .001$.

Besides, perception of program instructors also positively predicted perceived program effectiveness (Secondary 1: $\beta = .14$, $p < 0.001$; Secondary 2: $\beta = .20$, $p < 0.001$; Secondary 3: $\beta = .14$, $p < 0.001$; overall: $\beta = .15$, $p < 0.001$). These findings showed that subjective evaluation of program content and instructors were significant predictors of perceived effectiveness and they explained 35% of the variance in perceived program effectiveness across all the three grade levels of students.

Table 8. Multiple regression analyses predicting program effectiveness by program content and instructors

	Predictors			
	Program content	Program instructors	Model	
	ß[a]	ß[a]	R	R^2
S1	.48**	.14**	.59	.35
S2	.40**	.20**	.56	.31
S3	.49**	.14**	.60	.36
Overall	.47**	.15**	.59	.35

[a] Standardized coefficients. ** $p < .001$.

DISCUSSION

The present study examined the views of the students on the Tier 1 program of the community-based Project P.A.T.H.S. using the subjective outcome evaluation approach. Nearly 90% of the program participants returned the questionnaire, which covers perceived program content, instructors, and effectiveness. There are several strengths of the present study. First, the study employed a very large sample (N = 10,000+) which is rare in program evaluation studies. The large sample size helps make the statistical findings more stable and accurate. Second, the study employed validated instruments that had been tested repeatedly. The instruments showed good psychometric properties including test-retest reliability and construct validity (26-27). Third, the study examined the relationships amongst different aspects of client satisfaction and investigated how perceived program content and instructors predicted the overall perception of program effectiveness, which is not commonly examined in the evaluation literature. It demonstrated the usefulness of subjective outcome evaluation in accounting for program effectiveness and depicted the influence of different factors that could help build up models of outcome evaluation. Last but not least, this study examined the rating of satisfaction across different grade levels, which helped evaluate the applicability of the program to adolescents across three years of implementation.

The generally high satisfaction rate (over 85%) found in this study supported Hypothesis 1. This replicated the evaluation findings from both the Initial Implementation Phase and Extension Phase of the project (23-25). The program participants generally had very positive perception towards the program content, instructors, and program effectiveness, suggesting that the program was well-designed and delivered to the students in an adequate fashion. It is noteworthy that most of the participants perceived the program as effective in promoting different aspects of their development. Most of the participants (more than 75%) agreed that they would recommend the program to their friends and were willing to attend the program again. In short, the findings are generally in line with the previous studies (23-25). The consistent findings throughout the years suggested that adolescents had a favorable evaluation of the P.A.T.H.S. Program.

Amongst the three aspects of the evaluation, the participants reported the highest satisfaction rates in the program instructor domain. All the items under the aspect of instructor evaluation received more than 90% of satisfaction rate, implying that the instructors performed well in delivering the program. The findings give support to the effectiveness of the related training programs provided to the potential instructors (8, 25). The instructors had evaluated the training program that could enhance their self-confidence, self-reflection and efficacy in program delivery (8). Similarly, the results of the current study found that the students agreed the instructors had good performance such as mastery of the curriculum, good professional attitudes and teaching skills.

Regarding the inter-relationships amongst the three aspects of client satisfaction, Pearson correlation analyses found significant positive relationships. The findings support Hypotheses 2a, 2b and 2c. The results are generally consistent with previous studies in both initial implementation phase and extension phase (23-25), which found the program quality and program instructor to be closely associated. A possible explanation for this result may be that instructor qualities like mastery of the curriculum could predominantly decide the program content received by the students.

As for the differences amongst grades in subjective outcome ratings, the present findings are different from the previous studies (24-25). In the satisfaction ratings of program content and instructors, there was no significant difference amongst the three grades. The results are inconsistent with previous findings on subjective outcome evaluation (24-25), which found that younger students generally evaluated the program more positive in all aspects than did older students. However, the present study found significant grade differences in the evaluation of perceived program effectiveness and total effectiveness. Secondary 1 students evaluated the program as more effective than Secondary 2 and 3 students, where Secondary 2 students perceived the program as least effective. Regarding program effectiveness, the higher effectiveness reported by Secondary 1 students could be explained by their receptiveness to school involvement. Higher grade students were increasingly more susceptible to peer influence but less receptive to school involvement (28). They might be more critical and skeptical to what they learned while for younger students it may be easier to make changes simply for classroom learning. Of course, further research is needed to explain the contributing factors of grade difference in detail.

Consistent with our predictions (Hypothesis 4), multiple regression analyses showed that both perceived program quality and instructor quality were significant predictors of perceived program effectiveness. Results showed that the predictive power of perceived program quality and instructor quality was moderate amongst all the three grades (31-36%). The results are similar to former studies (25, 29). However, the current study could not replicate the high predictive power (more than 60%) found in other two earlier studies (23-24). Further studies are needed to explain the different findings as well as explore the factors interacting with program effectiveness.

In conclusion, the study showed that the program participants were overall satisfied with the Tier 1 program in all the three aspects of evaluation including program content, program instructors, and program effectiveness. Results also showed that perceived content and instructor quality could predict perceived program effectiveness. The major results of the study are consistent with previous studies (23-25) while attention should also be paid to the minor differences such as the grade difference found in perceived program effectiveness but not in perceived program content and instructor qualities. These new findings might imply the emerging needs of youth which consequently affect the applicability and effectiveness of PYD program.

Despite the positive results of the subjective outcome evaluation, the current study has several limitations. First, the data reported in this study were mainly from the quantitative part of client satisfaction evaluation. It would be helpful to further understand the in-depth learning experiences of the students. Second, behavioral changes such as improvement of peer relationship were not assessed in this study. It is suggested that additional evaluation effort should be made to evaluate the effectiveness of the program in the future, such as the use of objective outcome evaluation. Objective measures such as engagement in problem behaviors, academic performance, or participation in community services could be included in the future evaluation. Third, besides program content and instructors, other factors, which accounted for more than 60% of the variance in program effectiveness, were not covered in the study. As suggested by Chen (12), the characteristics of students and the learning environment may also affect program effectiveness. Group comparison studies could be employed to figure out other factors crucial to program effectiveness. Fourth, this study was a one-off cross-sectional evaluation study, which could not provide information about any long-term changes in the program participants. Further research such as longitudinal studies and case studies could be used to evaluate the changes of PYD qualities amongst the students. Despite the above limitations, the findings in this study still underline the effectiveness of the Tier 1 Program of the community-based P.A.T.H.S. Project based on the subjective outcome evaluation approach.

ACKNOWLEDGMENTS

The present paper and the Project P.A.T.H.S. are financially supported by The Hong Kong Jockey Club Charities Trust. The materials in this chapter are based on a paper published in the *International Journal on Disability and Human Development* 2017;16(4) issue.

REFERENCES

[1] Gottfredson DC, Wilson DB, Najaka SS. School-based crime prevention. In: Farrington DP, Sherman LW, Welsh B, Mackenzie DL, eds. *Evidence-based crime prevention.* London: Harwood Academic, 2002:56-164.

[2] Shek DTL. A review of validated youth prevention and positive youth development programs in Asia. Int J Adolesc Med Health 2011;23(4):317-24.

[3] Shek DTL. Adolescent developmental issues in Hong Kong: Relevance to positive youth development programs in Hong Kong. Int J Adolesc Med Health 2006;18 (3):341-54.

[4] Resnick MD, Ireland M, Borowsky I. Youth violence perpetration: What protects? What predicts? Findings from the National Longitudinal Study of Adolescent Health. J Adolesc Health 2004;35(424):1−10.

[5] Lösel F, Farrington DP. Direct protective and buffering protective factors in the development of youth violence. Am J Prev Med 2012;43(2):S8-23.

[6] Catalano RF, Berglund ML, Ryan J, Lonczak HS, Hawkins D. Positive youth development in the United States: Research findings on evaluations of positive youth development programs. Ann Am Acad Pol Soc Sci 2004;5:98-124.

[7] Shek DTL, Lee TY. Helping adolescents with greater psychosocial needs: Subjective outcome evaluation based on different cohorts. ScientificWorldJournal 2012; 694018:1-10. DOI: 10.1100/2012/694018.

[8] Shek DTL. Qualitative evaluation of the training program of the project P.A.T.H.S. in Hong Kong. Int J Adolesc Med Health 2010;22(3):425-35.

[9] Eccles J, Gootman J, eds. Community programs to promote youth development. Washington DC: National Academy Press, 2002.

[10] Grigoroudis E, Siskos Y. Customer satisfaction evaluation: Methods for measuring and implementing service quality. New York: Springer Science Business Media, 2010. DOI: 10.1007/978-1-4419-1640-2.

[11] Sabatelli RM, Anderson SA. Assessing outcomes in child and youth programs: A practical handbook, Rev. ed. Connecticut, CT: US Department of Justice to the State of Connecticut, 2005.

[12] Chen HT. Practical program evaluation: Assessing and improving planning, implementation, and effectiveness. Thousand Oaks, CA: Sage, 2005.

[13] Creemers BPM. From school effectiveness and school improvement to effective school improvement: Background, theoretical analysis, and outline of the empirical study. Educ Res Eval 2002;8:343-62.

[14] Mark E. Student satisfaction and the customer focus in higher education. J Higher Educ Policy Manag 2013;35:2-10.

[15] Lebow JL. Similarities and differences between mental health and health care evaluation studies assessing consumer satisfaction. Eval Program Plann 1983;6:237-45.

[16] Hill N, Roche G, Allen R. Customer satisfaction: The customer experience through the customer's eyes. London: Cogent Publishing, 2007.

[17] Fraser BJ. Research on classroom and school climate. In: Gabel D, ed. Handbook of research on science teaching and learning, New York: Macmillan, 1994:493–541.

[18] Rossi PH. Program outcomes: Conceptual measurement issues. In: Mullen EJ, Magnabosco JL, eds. Outcome measurement in the human services: Cross-cutting issues and methods. Washington, DC: NASW Press, 1997:20-34.

[19] Elliott KM. Key determinants of student satisfaction. J Coll Stud Ret 2003;4:271-79.

[20] Sweeney L. A predictive model of student satisfaction. Irish J Acad Prac 2016;5:1-30.

[21] Shek DTL. Subjective outcome and objective outcome evaluation findings: Insights from a Chinese context. Res Soc Work Prac 2010;20(3):293-301.

[22] Trotter C. What does client satisfaction tell us about effectiveness? Child Abuse Rev 2008;17:262-74.

[23] Shek DTL, Sun RCF. Participants' evaluation of the project P.A.T.H.S.: Are findings based on different datasets consistent? ScientificWorldJournal 2012;187450:1-9. DOI: 10.1100/2012/187450.

[24] Shek DTL, Law MYM. Evaluation of the Project P.A.T.H.S. based on the client satisfaction approach: View of the Students. J Pediatr Adolesc Gynecol 2014;27:S2-S9.

[25] Shek DTL, Ma CMS, Xie QZ. Evaluation of a community-based positive youth development program based on Chinese junior school students in Hong Kong. Int J Adolesc Med Health 2016;1-9. DOI: 10.1515/ijamh-2017-3002.

[26] Shek DTL, Ma CMS. Validation of a subjective outcome evaluation tool for participants in a positive youth development program in Hong Kong. J Pediatr Adolesc Gynecol 2014;27:S43-9.

[27] Yu L, Shek DTL. Testing factorial invariance across groups: An illustration using AMOS. Int J Disabil Hum Dev 2014;13:205-16.

[28] Sim TN, Koh SF. A domain conceptualization of adolescent susceptibility to peer pressure. J Res Adolescence 2003;13:57-80. DOI: 10.1111/1532-7795.1301002.

[29] Shek DTL, Ma CMS, Tang CYP. Predictors of subjective outcome evaluation findings in a positive youth development program in Hong Kong. Int J Disabil Hum Dev 2011;10(3): 249-55.

In: Soft Skills and Aspirations …
Editors: Daniel TL Shek, et al.
ISBN: 978-1-53614-092-7

Chapter 3

EVALUATION OF A COMMUNITY-BASED POSITIVE YOUTH DEVELOPMENT PROGRAM IN HONG KONG

Daniel TL Shek*[1-5,*]*, PhD, FHKPS, BBS, SBS, JP
and Xiaoqin Zhu*[1]*, PhD

[1]Department of Applied Social Sciences, The Hong Kong Polytechnic University, Hong Kong, PR China
[2]Centre for Innovative Programmes for Adolescents and Families, The Hong Kong Polytechnic University, Hong Kong, PR China
[3]Department of Social Work, East China Normal University, Shanghai, PR China
[4]Kiang Wu Nursing College of Macau, Macau, PR China
[5]Division of Adolescent Medicine, Department of Pediatrics, Kentucky Children's Hospital, University of Kentucky School of Medicine, Lexington, Kentucky, US

[*] Correspondence Author Email: daniel.shek@polyu.edu.hk.

ABSTRACT

Using the subjective outcome evaluation strategy, we investigated program implementers' perceptions of the Tier 1 Program of the community-based P.A.T.H.S. Project in Hong Kong. After completion of the program, 599 program implementers completed a valid and reliable scale (i.e., Form B) to give their ratings on program content, their own performance, and perceived program effectiveness. As expected, most program implementers perceived the program in a favorable way by giving very positive ratings on the three aspects measured in Form B. Grade differences on the ratings were observed, with implementers teaching the senior curriculum held more positive views on program effectiveness than did those teaching the junior curriculum. Similar to previous findings, perceived program content and perceived worker performance predicted program effectiveness. Findings of the present study provide further evidence for the success of the Tier 1 Program of the community-based P.A.T.H.S. Project in Hong Kong.

INTRODUCTION

It is well known around the world that school success is morbidly emphasized in Chinese societies. Because of the traditional Chinese belief that educational success leads to financial success and social status (1), Chinese students are expected by themselves and significant-others such as parents, teachers, and relatives to perform well in school and study hard to achieve high grades and academic excellence (2, 3). Such a strong emphasis on academic achievement is further intensified by the filial piety orientation in the collectivistic Chinese culture. Specifically, achieving school success is regarded as children's responsibility to their parents, and children's failure in school study may generate shame for the whole family (4). As a result, Chinese students usually experienced more academic stress than did their Western counterparts (5).

In Hong Kong, student performance at one learning stage determines their chance to study in an outstanding school in the following stage. Hence, students are struggling to survive and stand out in an educational environment characterized by intense competition and rigid selection, even early from kindergarten to higher education (6, 7). For example, students need to sit for public examinations prior to entering higher education. Although, the new "334" education schema (i.e., 3 years of junior secondary education, 3 years of senior secondary education and 4 years of undergraduate education) implemented since the academic year of 2009/2010 reduced the number of public examinations from two to one, the new secondary school curriculum posed extra challenges for adolescents. For example, "Liberal Studies" became a core subject (i.e., all students need to take this subject) under the new curriculum where students have to work much harder and exert extra effort (8).

With the above-mentioned circumstances, it is not surprising to find that over 45% of students regarded their studies as stressful, and even a larger proportion (i.e., 50.3%) of students felt pressure regarding the new curriculum (9). It is noteworthy that academic pressure experienced during adolescence can cause mental illness or other risk behavior. For example, a growing body of evidence suggested that academic pressure placed on adolescents was positively related to their anxiety and depression symptoms (3, 10, 11). Besides, school-related stress such as school performance felt by students during secondary school was positively associated with hopelessness (12), but inversely related to well-being (11, 12). An even serious consequence of the high level of academic stress was increased adolescent suicide ideation (13, 14). In fact, the time in a year when the number of suicide cases peaked paralleled with the examination periods, when there was a considerable increase in the academic stress of students (14).

Apart from the high level of pressure to excel in school, adolescents also face other challenges that result from pubertal change during adolescence. As a transitional phase from childhood to adulthood, adolescence is marked by a range of physiological, cognitive, psychological, emotional, and social changes, which could be potentially stressful (15). The stress resulting from these inevitable developmental changes makes adolescents especially vulnerable to develop a variety of problem behaviors, such as Internet addiction, substance abuse, sexual issues, school bullying, gambling, and delinquent acts. For example, 21.1% of secondary school adolescents in Iran showed problematic symptoms of Internet use (16). Among German students aged between 12 and 25 years, approximately 25%, 21%, and 6.4% of respondents reported current smoking, alcohol use, and cannabis use, respectively (17). In Taiwan, in a sample containing 2,119 youth aged 20 years, over 15% of them reported premarital sex experience when they were teenagers (18).

With respect to adolescent developmental problems in Hong Kong, researchers noted a rising and worrying trend of substance abuse, Internet addiction, premarital sex, school bullying, and material orientation (19). Recent studies revealed that the prevalence of these problem behaviors still remained at a high level. For example, Yu and Shek (20) reported that over one fifth of school adolescents displayed Internet addiction symptoms. In addition, Narcotics Division (21) showed that 2.3% of middle school students and 2.5% of post-secondary students took drugs. Although the percentage of Hong Kong adolescents attempting suicide (4%) was not high and was lower than the figures reported in other areas, quite a high proportion of adolescents manifested self-harm (22). In particular, research showed that more than 23% of junior secondary school students had ever engaged in deliberate self-harm behavior (e.g., direct cutting and scratching) in the past 12 months (22). This prevalence rate of self-harm is higher than that of mainland China adolescents, where nearly 17% committed self-harm during the past 12 months (23).

Considerable attention has been paid to adolescent problem behavior because of its high prevalence and significant negative influence on adolescent well-being and developmental outcomes. For example, Bradley and Greene (24) reviewed studies published between 1985 and 2010 to highlight associations between academic achievement and six types of risk behaviors in adolescents, including tobacco use, violence, drug (including alcohol) use, unprotected sexual activities, unhealthy dietary behaviors, and lack of physical activity. They found that 96.6% of the studies they reviewed reported significant and negative associations between adolescent risk behavior and academic performance. With the upsurge of adolescent problem behaviors and their long-standing negative impact on youth development (25), some scholars stated that it is especially important to promote adolescent positive youth development (PYD) attributes, which can help them maintain healthy functioning and cope with school distress and pubertal changes in an adaptive way (19, 26).

Different from traditional prevention approaches that focus on dealing with a single problem such as smoking or drinking, the PYD perspective highlights positive and bright sides of adolescents and regards adolescents as "resources to be developed" (27, p. 172). More specifically, the PYD approach emphasizes developmental assets and highlights adolescents' all-round healthy functioning in various domains, such as resilience, social and emotional competence, moral competence, and cognitive competence (28, 29). Accordingly, the aim of PYD programs is to prevent a variety of adolescent problems through promoting their positive development rather than to deal with one single problem at a time. The underlying philosophy is that adolescents will be less likely to develop problem behaviors if they are equipped with strong psychosocial competencies. This idea is similar to the belief in Chinese medicine - if the body is strong enough, symptoms of illness will not easily develop (19).

There is extensive evidence demonstrating that PYD programs are effective in strengthening adolescent competence and preventing adolescent risk behavior. For example, Catalano et al. (26) showed that well-evaluated universal, selective, and indicated PYD programs in different countries (e.g., USA, Australia, European countries, and Hong Kong) significantly enhanced participants' psychosocial competencies and educational attainment, while at the same time reduced their alcohol use, drug abuse, risky sexual activity, aggression and delinquency, crime, and depression. In Hong Kong, the most notable PYD program was the one entitled "Positive Adolescent Training through Holistic Social Programmes" (i.e., Project P.A.T.H.S.), which was designed by Shek and his collaborators to strengthen PYD qualities (i.e., multiple psychosocial competencies) in junior secondary school students (i.e., Grade 7 to 9) (30, 31).

The Project P.A.T.H.S. has two tiers of programs. The Tier 1 Program is a curricula-based universal program for students in all grade levels, and it was developed upon 15 PYD constructs (e.g., bonding, social and emotional competence, clear and positive identity, self-efficacy, and beliefs in the future) proposed by Catalano et al. (28) after reviewing the critical components of effective PYD programs. The Tier 2 Program is a selective program designed for those students with greater psychosocial needs, such as those students having family problems. With financial support from The Hong Kong Jockey Club Charities Trust, The Project P.A.T.H.S. has been successfully implemented from 2005/06 school year till present. From 2005/06 to 2011/12 school years, the project was implemented in the school context. A series of rigorous evaluation studies revealed a great success of the project as reflected by the high level of client satisfaction by different stakeholders, and enhanced competencies and reduced problem behaviors in the program participants (32-35).

Due to the remarkable success of the first seven years of implementation, the project was further transformed from a school-based mode to a community-based model commencing at 2013. In this phase, a number of non-governmental organizations (NGOs) providing service to children and youth were responsible for recruiting students and implementing the project. A community-based mode of PYD program implementation has its own strengths. For example, previous studies showed that implementation fidelity was higher in community-based contexts than that in a school-based model (36). One possible reason is that youth workers in communities such as social workers in NGOs may be more experienced than school teachers in implementing youth program materials. Besides, community-based delivery of the program will not be constrained by school time and arrangement of other courses or activities. As a result, programs run by NGOs can also involve students from schools that did not join the Project P.A.T.H.S., by inviting these students to apply by themselves.

According to existing evaluation studies (37-40), the first two years of community-based implementation of the Project P.A.T.H.S. was as effective as previous school-based implementation. To replicate these findings and to examine whether the third year (i.e., 2015) implementation was as smooth and effective as that in previous two years, we adopted the subjective outcome evaluation approach, which is also known as the client satisfaction approach to investigate program implementers' experience. Subjective outcome evaluation has been widely used in human service settings such as education, rehabilitation, counseling, and social work. This approach is convenient and efficient in revealing clients' views toward a program, which could further indicate the effectiveness of program implementation. Furthermore, some studies have shown that client satisfaction with the program was closely associated with findings of objective outcome evaluation, such as participant improvement in terms of enhanced PYD competencies (41, 42).

The present study focused on the Tier 1 Program of the Project P.A.T.H.S. implemented in 2015 by looking at program implementers' evaluation of the program, which could inform strengths, weaknesses, and directions of future improvement of the program (39). In previous studies, program implementers usually showed positive evaluations on the Tier 1 Program regarding the program content, their own performance, and program effectiveness (39, 43). In addition, program implementers' evaluation of program effectiveness could be significantly predicted by their perceptions of program content and their own performance. However, inconsistent findings were also reported in the area of grade differences in subjective outcome evaluation ratings. For example, Sun and Shek (43) found that implementers teaching junior students reported more positive evaluations in all aspects than did those teaching senior students. However, such a grade difference was not observed in other studies (39, 44). Based on these findings, the present study attempted to address the following questions and hypotheses:

How did implementers perceive the community-based Tier 1 Program implemented in 2015? Based on previous studies, positive evaluations were expected (H1).

Did implementers teaching different grades have different evaluations? Given the inconsistent findings in previous studies, we did not make specific hypotheses regarding this research question.

Were there any significant relationships among implementers' perceptions of program content, instructor performance, and effectiveness of the program? Based on previous findings, we hypothesized that evaluation of program effectiveness would be significantly related to program content (H2a) and implementers' performance (H2b). We also expected that program content (H3a) and implementers' performance (H3b) would be significant predictors of perceived effectiveness of the program.

OUR STUDY

In the third year of the community-based P.A.T.H.S. Project (i.e., 2015), there were 72 Tier 1 programs implemented by 21 agencies. Among these programs, 40, 18, and 13 were implemented at Secondary 1 (S1), Secondary 2 (S2), and Secondary 3 (S3) level respectively, with the remaining 1 program involving students from more than one grade. These programs were implemented by 713 teachers, social workers, and/or program workers, with 531, 108, and 73 implementers teaching S1, S2 and S3 curriculum respectively. The number of implementers across all programs ranged between 1 and 35, with a mean of 9.90 (SD = 7.61). Over half of the programs (n = 37, 51.39%) were taught by both teachers and social workers, while 44.44% (n = 32) of the programs were taught by social workers only and 3 programs (4.17%) were taught by teachers only. Regarding the implementation settings, a total of 65 programs (90.28%) were delivered in schools, while 4 programs (5.56%) were conducted in community centers and 3 programs (4.17%) were implemented in both settings.

Table 1. Reliability analyses and correlations among implementers' perceptions on different aspects

Subjective outcome evaluation scales	Cronbach's α	Mean inter-item correlation	Inter-scale correlation	
			Program content	Program implementers
Program content (10 items)	.92	.55	--	
Implementers' performance (10 items)	.93	.59	$.73^{***}$	
Program effectiveness (16 items)	.94	.52	$.55^{***}$	$.49^{***}$

*** $p < .001$

Table 2. Summary of the program implementers' positive perceptions toward the program content

	Respondents with positive responses (Options 4-6)							
	S1		S2		S3		Overall	
	n	%	*n*	%	*n*	%	*n*	%
1. The objectives of the curriculum are very clear.	443	97.6	78	97.5	63	98.4	585	97.7
2. The design of the curriculum is very good.	422	93.0	76	95.0	61	95.3	560	93.5
3. The activities were carefully planned.	430	94.7	77	96.3	63	98.4	571	95.3
4. The classroom atmosphere was very pleasant.	433	95.4	78	97.5	64	100.0	576	96.2
5. There was much peer interaction amongst the students.	426	93.8	79	98.8	62	96.9	568	94.8
6. Students participated actively during lessons (including discussions, sharing, games, etc.).	428	94.3	76	95.0	61	95.3	566	94.5
7. The program has a strong and sound theoretical support.	424	93.4	74	92.5	63	98.4	562	93.8
8. The teaching experience I encountered enhanced my interest towards the lessons.	416	91.6	73	91.3	62	96.9	552	92.2
9. Overall speaking, I have very positive evaluation of the program.	420	92.5	73	91.3	62	96.9	556	92.8
10. On the whole, students like this curriculum very much.	421	92.7	75	93.8	62	96.9	559	93.3

Note: All items were rated on a 6-point Likert scale with 1 = strongly disagree, 2 = disagree, 3 = slightly disagree, 4 = slightly agree, 5 = agree, 6 = strongly agree. Only respondents with positive responses (Options 4-6) are shown in the table.

S1: Secondary 1 level; S2: Secondary 2 level; S3: Secondary 3 level.

Table 3. Summary of the program implementers' positive perceptions toward their own performance

	Respondents with positive responses (Options 4-6)							
	S1		S2		S3		Overall	
	n	%	*n*	%	*n*	%	*n*	%
1. I have a good mastery of the curriculum.	436	96.0	78	97.5	62	96.9	577	96.3
2. I prepared well for the lessons.	436	96.0	78	97.5	63	98.4	578	96.5
3. My teaching skills were good.	437	96.3	78	97.5	64	100.0	580	96.8
4. I have good professional attitudes.	446	98.2	80	100.0	64	100.0	591	98.7
5. I was very involved.	444	97.8	79	98.8	64	100.0	588	98.2
6. I gained a lot during the course of instruction	422	93.0	76	95.0	60	93.8	559	93.3
7. I cared for the students.	448	98.7	80	100.0	64	100.0	593	99.0
8. I was ready to offer help to students when needed.	448	98.7	80	100.0	62	96.9	591	98.7
9. I had much interaction with the students.	436	96.0	78	97.5	62	96.9	577	96.3
10. Overall speaking, I have very positive evaluation of myself as an instructor.	445	98.0	78	97.5	64	100.0	588	98.2

Note: All items were reported on a 6-point Likert scale with 1 = strongly disagree, 2 = disagree, 3 = slightly disagree, 4 = slightly agree, 5 = agree, 6 = strongly agree. Only respondents with positive responses (Options 4-6) are shown in the table.
S1: Secondary 1 level; S2: Secondary 2 level; S3: Secondary 3 level.

To evaluate the effectiveness of the Tier 1 Program, program implementers were invited to respond to a scale named as "Subjective Outcome Evaluation Form for Instructors" (i.e., Form B) after completion of the program. A total of 599 implementers completed Form B, resulting in an overall response rate of 82.99%. An evaluation manual with detail guidelines on collection and analyses of Form B data were given to the implementers.

Table 4. Summary of the program implementers' positive perceptions toward the program effectiveness

		Respondents with positive responses (Options 3-5)							
		S1		S2		S3		Overall	
		n	%	*n*	%	*n*	%	*n*	%
1.	It has strengthened students' bonding with teachers, classmates and their families.	425	93.6	74	92.5	60	93.8	560	93.5
2.	It has strengthened students' resilience in adverse conditions.	436	96.0	73	91.3	63	98.4	573	95.7
3.	It has enhanced students' social competence.	446	98.2	76	95.0	63	98.4	586	97.8
4.	It has improved students' ability in handling and expressing emotions.	439	96.7	74	92.5	62	96.9	576	96.2
5.	It has enhanced students' cognitive competence.	430	94.7	74	92.5	62	96.9	567	94.7
6.	Students' ability to resist harmful influences has been improved.	428	94.3	73	91.3	60	93.8	562	93.8
7.	It has strengthened students' ability to distinguish between the good and the bad.	442	97.4	77	96.3	61	95.3	581	97.0
8.	It has increased students' competence in making sensible and wise choices.	439	96.7	73	91.3	62	96.9	575	96.0
9.	It has helped students to have life reflections.	415	91.4	71	88.8	60	93.8	547	91.3
10.	It has reinforced students' self-confidence.	429	94.5	76	95.0	64	100.0	570	95.2
11.	It has increased students' self-awareness.	440	96.9	77	96.3	64	100.0	582	97.2
12.	It has helped students to face the future with a positive attitude.	432	95.2	77	96.3	63	98.4	573	95.7
13.	It has helped students to cultivate compassion and care about others.	423	93.2	73	91.3	59	92.2	556	92.8
14.	It has encouraged students to care about the community.	396	87.2	65	81.3	55	85.9	517	86.3
15.	It has promoted students' sense of responsibility in serving the society.	400	88.1	67	83.8	53	82.8	521	87.0
16.	It has enriched the overall development of the students.	437	96.3	76	95.0	64	100.0	578	96.5

Note: All items were reported on a 5-point Likert scale with 1 = unhelpful, 2 = not very helpful, 3 = slightly helpful, 4 = helpful, 5 = very helpful. Only respondents with positive responses (Options 3-5) are shown in the table.

S1: Secondary 1 level; S2: Secondary 2 level; S3: Secondary 3 level.

Instruments

The Form B used in the current study was a valid and reliable measure and has been widely used in previous evaluation studies (41, 44). This measure consisted of both quantitative and qualitative questions. However, the present study only focused on quantitative data due to space limitation. Quantitative questions assessed implementers' views via three subscales: program content (10 items), implementer performance (10 items), and program effectiveness (16 items). As shown in table 1, these three subscales had good reliability in the present study with Cronbach's α above .90. In addition to these three subscales, three other items measured implementers' willingness to suggest other students to join the program (1 item), willingness to work as instructors in similar programs in future (1 item), and the extent to which the program was helpful for personal growth (1 item). For subscales of program content and implementer performance, a 6-point scale was used while a 5-point scale was adopted for program effectiveness subscale. For all items, higher scores indicated more positive evaluations.

Data analyses

In the present study, individual data of the implementers were used as basic units of analysis. Firstly, we performed reliability analyses for the three subscales (i.e., program content, implementers' performance, and program effectiveness) of Form B. Then, descriptive statistical analyses were carried out to indicate the percentage of positive responses regarding implementer perceptions of different aspects of the Tier 1 Program. To examine differences in implementers' evaluations across different grade levels, a multivariate analysis of variance (MANOVA) was further conducted, with grade as the independent variable and implementers' evaluations on three subscales as dependent variables. Correlations amongst implementers' evaluations on different aspects of the program were investigated using Pearson correlation analyses. Several multiple regression analyses were conducted to examine whether evaluations of program content and program implementers' performance significantly predicted perceived program effectiveness across the three grade levels.

OUR FINDINGS

Numbers and percentages of implementers having positive evaluations of the Tier 1 Program on the different domains of the scale are shown in table 2 to 5. Overall speaking, implementers had positive evaluations on all aspects. As a result, Hypothesis 1 was supported. As shown in table 2, implementers' views toward program content were overall positive, with over 90% of the implementers giving positive ratings on all the ten items across all grade levels. In addition, most implementers agreed that "the design of the curriculum is very good" (93.5%) and "the classroom atmosphere was very pleasant" (96.2%), and 92.8% of the implementers had very positive views of the program. For implementers' own performance, most implementers also reported favorable evaluations (see Table 3). More specifically, 98.2% of implementers had very positive evaluations of themselves, and 99% of them thought that they cared for the students, and over 98% of implementers regarded themselves as "having good professional attitudes", "very involved", and "ready to offer help to students when needed".

Similar positive results were found for the perceived effectiveness of the program. As demonstrated in table 4, more than 96% of implementers endorsed that the program promoted students' overall development. Most implementers also indicated that the program strengthened students' resilience (95.7%), social competence (97.8%), ability to distinguish good and bad (97.0%), and competence in making wise choices (96.0%). Table 5 shows implementers' ratings on the additional three questions. Over 90% of the participants indicated that they were willing to suggest other students to participate in the program (94.8%) and teach similar programs in future (93.2%). Besides, nearly 95% of the implementers thought the program helped promote their personal growth.

Table 5. Summary of the program implementers' positive perceptions toward other aspects

Items	S1		S2		S3		Overall	
	n	%	*n*	%	*n*	%	*n*	%
[a] Willingness to suggest other students to participate in the program	428	94.3	75	93.8	64	100	568	94.8
[a] Willingness to teach similar programs in future	418	92.1	77	96.3	62	96.9	558	93.2
[b] The extent to which the program helped implementers' personal growth	424	93.4	77	96.3	62	96.9	564	94.2

Note: S1: Secondary 1 level; S2: Secondary 2 level; S3: Secondary 3 level.
a: A 4-point Likert scale was used, with 1 = definitely will not, 2 = will not, 3 = will, 4 = definitely will. Only respondents with positive responses (Options 3-4) are shown in the table.
b: A 5-point Likert scale was used, with 1 = unhelpful, 2 = not very helpful, 3 = slightly helpful, 4 = helpful, 5 = very helpful. Only respondents with positive responses (Options 3-5) are shown in the table.

The results of MANOVA are depicted in table 6. Grade differences were not observed for implementers' evaluations of program content and their own performance. However, a significant grade difference was found for perceived program effectiveness (F (2, 573) = 5.06, p = .007, η^2_p = .02). Post-hoc analyses revealed that implementers teaching Secondary 3 students (M = 3.93, SD = .53) perceived higher program effectiveness than did those teaching Secondary 1 students (M = 3.69, SD = .55, p = .005).

Table 6. Comparisons of implementers' subjective outcome evaluation on different aspects across grades

	S1 (n = 437)		S2 (n = 76)		S3 (n = 63)		MANOVA	
	M	*SD*	*M*	*SD*	*M*	*SD*	*F*	$p\eta^2$
Program content (10 items)	4.70	.60	4.73	.56	4.84	.43	1.92	.007
Implementers' performance (10 items)	4.85	.57	4.91	.48	5.02	.49	2.72	.009
Program effectiveness (16 items)	3.69	.55	3.74	.54	3.93	.53	5.06**	.017

Note: S1: Secondary 1 level; S2: Secondary 2 level; S3: Secondary 3 level. ** p < .01.

Table 7. Multiple regression analyses predicting perceived program effectiveness by perceptions on program content and implementers' performance

	β		F	R^2
	Program content	Implementers' performance		
Secondary 1	.40***	.21***	101.48***	.32
Secondary 2	.61***	.01	22.01***	.36
Secondary 3	.32*	.25	11.37***	.25
Overall	.42***	.19***	137.59***	.32

* $p < .05$; *** $p < .001$.

The correlation coefficients among evaluations of program content, performance of the implementers, and effectiveness of the program are shown in table 1. Consistent with our hypotheses (i.e., H2a and H2b), program content quality ($r = .55, p < .001$) and implementer performance ($r = .49, p < .001$) were both positively associated with perceived program effectiveness. According to multiple regression analyses (see table 7), both perceived program content ($\beta = .40, p < .001$) and worker performance ($\beta = .21, p < .001$) were significant predictors of perceived program effectiveness at Secondary 1 level. However, only perceived program content significantly predicted perceived program effectiveness at Secondary 2 ($\beta = .61, p < .001$) and Secondary 3 ($\beta = .32, p < .05$) levels, whereas worker performance did not have significant predicting effect at these two grade levels. For the whole dataset, both evaluations of program content ($\beta = .42, p < .001$) and implementer performance ($\beta = .19, p < .001$) significantly predicted perceived program effectiveness. This overall model accounted for 32% of the variance of perceived program effectiveness. As a result, Hypothesis 3a was supported at each grade level and whole dataset, while Hypothesis 3b was supported at Secondary 1 level and the whole sample.

DISCUSSION

The present research attempted to replicate previous evaluation findings regarding implementers' perceptions of the Tier 1 Program of the community-based Project P.A.T.H.S. in Hong Kong. To do this, the present study utilized a valid and reliable measure of subjective outcome evaluation to assess the implementers' views on several aspects, including program content, implementer performance, program effectiveness, willingness to recommend the program to other students, willingness to teach similar programs in future, and whether the implementation experience helped promote implementers' personal growth. These measures not only helped explore implementers' evaluation in a comprehensive way, but also allowed us to further clarify the factors contributing to perceived program effectiveness. Besides, a large sample was used in the present study (n = 599), which enhanced the generalizability of present findings to the populations.

Overall speaking, for the community-based Tier 1 Program implemented in 2015, the implementers held positive perceptions of the program. For example, the implementers perceived the program content positively: approximately 98% of them considered that curriculum objectives were clear; nearly 94% perceived the curriculum was well designed; and over 95% agreed that the activities were meticulously designed. Besides, the implementers held favorable views toward their own performance. Over 95% of the program implementers regarded themselves as caring, willing to help students and well prepared for the lessons. These findings are largely in line with previous evaluation findings (39, 44).

The implementers also perceived the Tier 1 Program as effective in promoting different areas of development in the students, including resilience, social competence, cognitive competence, self-awareness, social responsibility, and ability in distinguishing good and bad. Noteworthy, most implementers (over 90%) were willing to suggest other students to join the program and teach similar programs in future, and nearly 95% of the implementers thought the program increased their personal growth. Together with previous findings (38, 39), the positive results found in the present study suggest that the Project P.A.T.H.S. is quite successful in Hong Kong no matter in which context (i.e., school or community) it is implemented. As the increase in adolescents' positive youth development (PYD) qualities would promote adaptability and well-being as well as reduce adolescent problem behaviors (9, 45, 46), the Project P.A.T.H.S. with an objective to promote adolescents' PYD competencies is regarded as a timely and effective means of minimizing negative influences of high academic pressure and extensive developmental challenges on Hong Kong adolescents.

In the current study, we did not find grade differences in implementers' evaluations of program content and their own performance. These results are in line with most of the previous studies which also did not find grade differences in implementers' subjective outcome evaluation (39, 44). The results suggest that programs for all grades were well designed and all implementers were well engaged regardless of intended grades. However, one unique finding in the present study was that implementers teaching senior form (i.e., Secondary 3 level) rated the program as more effective than did implementers teaching junior form (i.e., Secondary 1 level). This result is quite different from previous findings, in that some studies found similar ratings for program effectiveness among implementers in different grades (39, 44), and one study found lower ratings for program effectiveness among implementers in senior grades compared with perceived program effectiveness in junior grades (43). On one hand, the present finding suggests that students in senior grades were not necessarily less interested in and worse engaged in the program, just as some studies found that students in higher grades had better perceptions of PYD programs than did students in lower grades (40). On the other hand, as numbers of implementers in different grades varied a lot, and the sample size of the present study was smaller than that of Sun and Shek's (43) study, the present finding needs to be replicated in future studies using a larger sample size and more balanced sub-samples in different grades.

Theories and empirical studies suggested that there were five salient factors contributing to the effectiveness of PYD programs: program, people, policy, place, and process (i.e., 5P model) (47). The present study considered two factors: "program" (i.e., program content) and "people" (i.e., implementers). Congruent with this 5P model and similar to previous studies (44), the present study showed that evaluations on program content and implementer performance were both positively associated with perceived program effectiveness. These findings supported Hypotheses 2a and 2b. In addition, multiple regression analyses indicated that both evaluations of program content and worker performance were significant predictors of perceived program effectiveness in the whole sample. Hence, Hypothesis 3a and Hypothesis 3b were also supported. However, perceived program content significantly predicted perceived program effectiveness in all grade levels, while perceived implementer quality only showed significant effect on Secondary 1 grade. One possible reason may be due to the small sub-sample size on Secondary 2 and 3 grades. Hence, further research with a larger sample size at each grade level is in need to elucidate the present finding.

The current study has several limitations. First, although subjective outcome evaluation approach has its own advantages, it suffers from inherent limitations, such as systematic biases result from item order, psychological factors and macroeconomic fluctuations (48). Therefore, findings should be interpreted with caution, and future studies could include both objective and subjective measures to test program effectiveness. Second, the present study was quantitative in nature. Qualitative designs such as focus group interview should be further included to present a more comprehensive picture of the Project P.A.T.H.S. implemented in the community contexts. Lastly, only two factors (i.e., program and people) of the 5P model were considered as potential predictors of program effectiveness in the present study. Thus, it is hard to identify other contributing factors and explore interactions among these factors. It will certainly be illuminating to take into account more factors that would affect program success.

Despite these limitations, the present study showed that program implementers were highly satisfied with the Tier 1 Program of the Project P.A.T.H.S. implemented based on the community contexts in 2015. More specifically, both program content and implementers' performance got extremely good ratings. In addition, the program implementers perceived that both students and they themselves benefited a lot from the program. Together with previous evaluation findings, the present study again suggests that the Project P.A.T.H.S. can effectively promote holistic development in Hong Kong adolescents.

ACKNOWLEDGMENTS

The present paper and the Project P.A.T.H.S. are financially supported by the Hong Kong Jockey Club Charities Trust. The materials in this chapter are based on a paper published in the *International Journal on Disability and Human Development* 2017;16(4) issue.

REFERENCES

[1] Hesketh T, Ding QJ. Anxiety and depression in adolescents in urban and rural China. Psychol Rep 2005;96:435-44.

[2] Shek DTL, Chan LK. Hong Kong Chinese parents' perceptions of the ideal child. J Psychol 1999;133:291-302.

[3] Quach AS, Epstein NB, Riley PJ, Falconier MK, Fang X. Effects of parental warmth and academic pressure on anxiety and depression symptoms in Chinese adolescents. J Child Fam Stud 2015;24:106-16.

[4] Triandis HC, McCusker C, Hui CH. Multimethod probes of individualism and collectivism. J Pers Soc Psychol 1990;59:1006-20.

[5] Liu Y, Lu Z. The Chinese high school student's stress in the school and academic achievement. Educ Psychol 2011;31:27-35.

[6] Kwan YK. Life satisfaction and self-assessed health among adolescents in Hong Kong. J Happiness Stud 2010;11:383-93.

[7] Jaffee D. The general education initiative in Hong Kong: Organized contradictions and emerging tensions. High Educ 2012;64:193-206.

[8] Chan CK, Luk LY. Faculty perspectives on the "3+ 3+ 4" curriculum reform in Hong Kong: A case study. Int Educ Stud 2013;6:56-66.

[9] Shek DTL, Leung H. Perceived family quality of life, school competence, and academic adjustment among early adolescents in Hong Kong. In: Shek DTL, Sun RCF, Ma CMS, eds. Chinese Adolescents in Hong Kong. Singapore: Springer, 2014:71-91.

[10] Liu Y, Lu Z. Chinese high school students' academic stress and depressive symptoms: Gender and school climate as moderators. Stress Health 2012;28:340-6.

[11] Moksnes UK, Løhre A, Lillefjell M, Byrne DG, Haugan G. The association between school stress, life satisfaction and depressive symptoms in adolescents: Life satisfaction as a potential mediator. Soc Indic Res 2016;125:339-57.

[12] Shek DTL, Li X. Perceived school performance, life satisfaction, and hopelessness: A 4-year longitudinal study of adolescents in Hong Kong. Soc Indic Res 2016;126:921-34.

[13] Ang RP, Huan VS. Relationship between academic stress and suicidal ideation: Testing for depression as a mediator using multiple regression. Child Psychiatr Hum Dev 2006;37:133-43.

[14] Ung EK. Youth suicide and parasuicide in Singapore. Ann Acad Med Singapore 2003;32:12-8.

[15] Moksnes UK, Byrne DG, Mazanov J, Espnes GA. Adolescent stress: Evaluation of the factor structure of the adolescent stress questionnaire (ASQ-N). Scand J Psychol 2010;51:203-9.

[16] Ahmadi K, Saghafi A. Psychosocial profile of Iranian adolescents' Internet addiction. Cyberpsychol Behav Soc Netw 2013;16:543-8.

[17] Walther B, Morgenstern M, Hanewinkel R. Co-occurrence of addictive behaviours: Personality factors related to substance use, gambling and computer gaming. Eur Addict Res 2012;18:167-74.

[18] Chiao C, Yi C-C, Ksobiech K. Exploring the relationship between premarital sex and cigarette/alcohol use among college students in Taiwan: A cohort study. BMC Public Health 2012;12:527-36.

[19] Shek DTL, Keung Ma H, Sun RCF. A brief overview of adolescent developmental problems in Hong Kong. ScientificWorldJournal 2011;11:2243-56.

[20] Yu L, Shek DTL. Internet addiction in Hong Kong adolescents: A three-year longitudinal study. J Pediatr Adolesc Gynecol 2013;26:S10-7.

[21] Narcotics Division, Security Bureau. The 2014/15 survey of drug use among students. URL: http://www.nd.gov.hk/en/survey_of_drug_use_14-15.htm.

[22] Law BMF, Shek DTL. Self-harm and suicide attempts among young Chinese adolescents in Hong Kong: Prevalence, correlates, and changes. J Pediatr Adolesc Gynecol 2013;26:S26-32.

[23] Wan Y-H, Hu C-L, Hao J-H, Sun Y, Tao F-B. Deliberate self-harm behaviors in Chinese adolescents and young adults. Eur Child Adolesc Psychiatr 2011;20:517-25.

[24] Bradley BJ, Greene AC. Do health and education agencies in the United States share responsibility for academic achievement and health? A review of 25 years of evidence about the relationship of adolescents' academic achievement and health behaviors. J Adolesc Health 2013;52:523-32.

[25] Pergamit MR, Huang L, Lane J. The long-term impact of adolescent risky behaviors and family environment. URL: http://aspe.hhs.gov/execsum/long-term-impact-adolescent-risky-behaviors-and-family-environment

[26] Catalano RF, Fagan AA, Gavin LE, Greenberg MT, Irwin CE, Ross DA, et al. Worldwide application of prevention science in adolescent health. Lancet 2012;379:1653-64.

[27] Lerner RM, Dowling EM, Anderson PM. Positive youth development: Thriving as the basis of personhood and civil society. Appl Dev Sci 2003;7:172-80.

[28] Catalano RF, Berglund ML, Ryan JA, Lonczak HS, Hawkins JD. Positive youth development in the United States: Research findings on evaluations of positive youth development programs. Ann Am Acad Polit Soc Sci 2004;591:98-124.

[29] Lerner RM, Liberty: Thriving and civic engagement among American youth, 1st ed. Thousand Oaks, CA: Sage, 2004.

[30] Shek DTL, Sun RCF. The Project P.A.T.H.S. in Hong Kong: Development, training, implementation, and evaluation. J Pediatr Adolesc Gynecol 2013;26:S2-9.

[31] Shek DTL, Sun RCF, editors. Development and evaluation of Positive Adolescent Training through Holistic Social Programs (P.A.T.H.S.). Singapore: Springer, 2013.

[32] Shek DTL, Ma CMS. Impact of the Project PATHS in the junior secondary school years: Individual growth curve analyses. ScientificWorldJournal 2011;11:253-66.

[33] Shek DTL, Yu L. Impact of the Project PATHS on adolescent risk behavior: A five-year longitudinal study. In: Shek DTL, Sun RCF, editors. Development and evaluation of Positive Adolescent Training through Holistic Social Programs (P.A.T.H.S.). Singapore: Springer, 2013:85-106.

[34] Shek DTL, Sun RCF. Positive youth development programs for adolescents with greater psychosocial needs: Subjective outcome evaluation over 3 years. J Pediatr Adolesc Gynecol 2014;27:S17-25.

[35] Shek DTL, Yu L, Ho VYT. Subjective outcome evaluation and factors related to perceived effectiveness of the Project P.A.T.H.S. in Hong Kong. ScientificWorldJournal 2012;2012:Article 490290.

[36] Fagan AA, Hanson K, Hawkins JD, Arthur MW. Implementing effective community-based prevention programs in the Community Youth Development Study. Youth Violence Juv Justice 2008;6:256-78.

[37] Shek DTL, Zhu X, Wu FKY. Subjective outcome evaluation of the community-based program of the P.A.T.H.S. project in Hong Kong. Int J Child Adolesc Health 2017;10:139-51.

[38] Shek DTL, Liang RLY, Ma CMS. Subjective outcome evaluation of the community-based project P.A.T.H.S. in Hong Kong. Int J Child Adolesc Health 2017;10:115-25.

[39] Shek DTL, Ng CSM, Law MYM. Community-based positive youth development program in Hong Kong: views of the program implementers. Int J Adolesc Med Health 2017;29:15-21.

[40] Shek DTL, Law MYM. Evaluation of programs for adolescents with greater psychosocial needs: Community-based P.A.T.H.S. Project in Hong Kong. Int J Adolesc Med Health 2017;29:23-31.

[41] Shek DTL. Is subjective outcome evaluation related to objective outcome evaluation? Insights from a longitudinal study in Hong Kong. J Pediatr Adolesc Gynecol 2014;27:S50-6.
[42] Shek DTL. Subjective outcome and objective outcome evaluation findings: Insights from a Chinese context. Res Soc Work Pract 2010;20:293-301.
[43] Sun RCF, Shek DTL. Perceived program qualities and outcomes of a youth program in Hong Kong based on the views of the workers. J Pediatr Adolesc Gynecol 2014;27:S10-6.
[44] Shek DTL, Pu EX, Leung JTY, Law MYM. Subjective outcome evaluation of the community-based P.A.T.H.S. project: Views of program implementers. Int J Child Adolesc Health 2017;10:127-37.
[45] Sun RCF, Shek DTL. Longitudinal influences of positive youth development and life satisfaction on problem behaviour among adolescents in Hong Kong. Soc Indic Res 2013;114:1171-97.
[46] Shek DTL, Liang J. Risk factors and protective factors in substance abuse in Chinese adolescents in Hong Kong. In: Lee TY, Shek DTL, Sun RCF, eds. Student well-being in Chinese adolescents in Hong Kong: Theory, intervention and research. Singapore: Springer, 2015:237-53.
[47] Shek DTL, Sun RCF. Implementation of a positive youth development program in a Chinese context: The role of policy, program, people, process, and place. ScientificWorldJournal 2008;8:980-96.
[48] Jahedi S, Méndez F. On the advantages and disadvantages of subjective measures. J Econ Behav Organ 2014;98:97-114.

In: Soft Skills and Aspirations … ISBN: 978-1-53614-092-7
Editors: Daniel TL Shek, et al.

Chapter 4

EVALUATION OF A COMMUNITY-BASED POSITIVE YOUTH DEVELOPMENT PROGRAM FOR ADOLESCENTS WITH GREATER PSYCHOSOCIAL NEEDS

Daniel TL Shek*[1-5,*], *PhD, FHKPS, BBS, JP,
Cecilia MS Ma*[1], *PhD and Peixuan Zhao*[1], *MA
[1]Department of Applied Social Sciences,
The Hong Kong Polytechnic University, Hong Kong, PR China
[2]Centre for Innovative Programmes for Adolescents and Families,
The Hong Kong Polytechnic University, Hong Kong, PR China
[3]Department of Social Work, East China Normal University,
Shanghai, PR China
[4]Kiang Wu Nursing College of Macau, Macau, PR China
[5]Division of Adolescent Medicine, Department of Pediatrics,
Kentucky Children's Hospital,
University of Kentucky School of Medicine, Lexington,
Kentucky, US

---

[*] Corresponding Author Email: daniel.shek@polyu.edu.hk.

ABSTRACT

In this chapter, we attempt to investigate the perceptions of Chinese secondary school students with greater psychosocial needs of the Tier 2 Program in the community-based phase of the P.A.T.H.S. Project in Hong Kong (N = 4,245). Using a subjective outcome evaluation tool (Form C), results revealed that great majority of the students held positive attitudes toward the program, implementers and the effectiveness of the program. Also, the three domains of the program ("program quality," "implementer quality" and "program effectiveness") were significantly associated with each other. In line with previous findings, both program content and program implementer quality were significant predictors of program effectiveness. The current findings further reinforce the thesis that the community-based Tier 2 programs of the P.A.T.H.S. Project are effectiveness in promoting the holistic development of adolescents with greater psychosocial needs in Hong Kong.

INTRODUCTION

Adolescents are typically at risk for engaging in developmental problems including substance abuse, criminal behavior, mental health, and unhealthy lifestyle such as underage smoking, drinking and moral issues (1, 2). Such developmental problems adversely affect adolescent development on multiple levels, including physical, psychological, emotional, social and spiritual domains, which may eventually adversely affect social stability (3).

For instance, bullying behavior in school is a widespread problem with roughly 25%-30% of students involved in bullying in each school year (4). A national study among US adolescents showed that the prevalence of having bullied others or having been bullied physically, verbally, socially, and electronically at school for at least once in the last 2 months was 20.8%, 53.6%, 51.4% and 13.6%, respectively (5). Besides, cyberbullying or electronic bullying is emerging with the rapid development of technology (6, 7). After reviewing 35 articles in this field, research showed that approximately 24% of youth had been cyberbullied (8). In recent years, researchers have demonstrated many harmful effects of bullying on adolescent school achievement, pro-social skills and psychological wellbeing (9, 10). Previous research also found that risk factors for being bullied included poor academic achievement, unhealthy friendship and peer relationships, bad communication with parents, and being isolated (11). Furthermore, youths who were victimized were at a greater risk of developing psychosocial and internalizing problems (12). Particularly, cyber bullying victims were more likely to be isolated, felt hopeless and reported severe depressive symptoms (13). Recognizing these complex and urgent problems, various school-based programs using different prevention approaches have been developed to reduce bullying and other aggressive behaviors among adolescents. A recent systematic meta-analytic review of anti-bullying programs evaluation in school showed that the average reduction in bullying and victimization in these programs was 20-23% (14).

Another example of adolescent developmental issues is substance abuse. Results from a national comorbidity adolescent survey found that alcohol and drug use were quite common in US, with 78.2% of adolescents consuming alcohol and about 16.4% taking illicit drug abuse (15). A study using meta-analysis to examine the effectiveness of drug treatment programs showed that although most types of treatment had short-term effect in reducing substance abuse, smaller long-term improvement outcomes were reported (16). Turning to Hong Kong, based on the result of students' drug use survey released in 2015 by the Narcotics Division of the Hong Kong Special Administrative Government, although there was a drop in lifetime prevalence in drug-taking amongst students, 0.7%, 2.2% and 2.5% of students in upper primary, secondary and post-secondary levels reported to have abused drugs, respectively. Moreover, the number of abusers of cannabis increased to 59.1%. Compared with the results of survey in 2011, most of adolescent abusers (80.9%) still never sought help from others (17).

In view of the existing adolescent developmental problems, minimizing the occurrence of adolescent problem behaviors and helping them develop in a healthy manner is of critical importance. An alternative approach, which is different from the past that centers on pathologies and problems of adolescents, has been proposed with focus on addressing positive youth development (PYD) (18). PYD emphasizes discovering and developing adolescents' talents, strengths, future potentials and interests (19). As a strategy to facilitate the healthy growth of youth development and positive health outcomes, the support for PYD has been endorsed by the Division of Reproductive Health at the Disease Control and Prevention Centers in US (20).

In the process of becoming an adult, youth developmental challenges include identity formation, career exploration, and increased social responsibility. Hence, programs should be designed to meet adolescent developmental needs and promote their psychosocial competences (21). Through a review of 77 existing PYD programs, Catalano et al. (22) identified 15 PYD constructs that were commonly covered in successful PYD programs. These constructs included "bonding, resilience, social competence, recognition of positive behavior, emotional competence, cognitive competence, behavioral competence, moral competence, self-determination, self-efficacy, clear and positive identity, beliefs in the future, prosocial involvement, prosocial norms, and spirituality."

While PYD programs were built and implemented in the West (23), literature review revealed that systematic, multi-years, and evidence-based PYD programs are lacking in Hong Kong (24). Against this background, using the 15 PYD constructs as the conceptual framework, a multi-year project entitled Positive Adolescent Training through Holistic Social Programmes (Project P.A.T.H.S.) was launched in 2005. The project was funded by The Hong Kong Jockey Club Charities Trust (HK$400 million) in collaboration with the Research Team, the Education Bureau (formerly Education and Manpower Bureau) and the Social Welfare Department. With the involvement of roughly half of the Hong Kong secondary schools, this PYD programs has been successfully implemented since 2005/2006 school year, with very encouraging evaluation findings (25). From 2009/2010 school year, the HKCCT earmarked additional funding (HK$350 million) to further promote a three-year extension of the P.A.T.H.S. Project.

One unique feature of this PYD project is that several evaluation methods have been applied to examine the impact of the project (26). Various evaluative strategies have been used to examine the project, including subjective outcome evaluation based on program participants and program implementers, objective outcome evaluation, qualitative evaluation, process evaluation, classroom observations, repertory grid tests and student products such as students' weekly diaries and drawings (27). According to the results from eight waves of data collected over five consecutive years, the program showed positive impact in promoting youth holistic development and preventing youth problem behaviors (28). With the great success in school-based program, a community-based project was implemented in 2013 lasting until the end of 2017.

The P.A.T.H.S. Project consists of two tiers of programs. Based on a systematic, evidence-based and comprehensive curriculum that normally provides 10 to 20 hours training for the students each year, the Tier 1 program is developed for Secondary 1 to 3 students. The Tier 2 program is developed for students in each grade with greater psychosocial needs (27). As previous research on bullying intervention programs suggested that victimization are mainly influenced by parents and friends (6) and that programs with parental involvement are more effective (29), programs involving parents are also designed. Hence, participants of community-based Tier 2 program are different from that of school-based programs. In the past years, while students, implementers and parents were involved in some programs, there were some programs only engaged students or both students and implementers.

It is noteworthy that under the community-based phase, non-governmental organizations (NGOs) were also involved in the Tier 2 program. The NGOs took the responsibility to plan the most appropriate programs to meet participants' needs. Previous studies showed that changing of social systems could successfully affect adolescents (29). In the community-based phase, different programs aiming to strengthen adolescent psychosocial competence were developed (30). Generally speaking, various program modes were developed in the Tier 2 Program. These included "adventure-based counseling programs" (ABC), "voluntary training and service programs" (VTS), programs with both ABC and VTS elements, and programs with other elements such as parental involvement (31). Results of data analyses of 153,761 students in previous Tier 2 programs suggested that most of the students regarded the program as successful in promoting their holistic development (25).

To replicate the previous findings and to examine program effectiveness among participants in the community-based implementation phase, the subjective outcome evaluation approach was used to examine participants' views of the program. As an economical and efficient tool, subjective outcome evaluation is commonly used to investigate client satisfaction (32). Typically, participants are asked questions including "whether they are satisfied with the program and whether they perceive the program to be beneficial to them." To assess the influence of different aspects of the program (such as implementers' qualities, content, time arrangement and effectiveness of the program) on participants' perceptions, client satisfaction scales with different dimensions were used (33). Previous research showed that reports completed by the program implementers could reveal program effectiveness (34). Besides, objective outcome and subjective outcome ratings were significantly correlated.

In this study, a subjective outcome evaluation scale (Form C) was given to the students after completing the whole program. In previous studies, the factor structure and reliability of Form C were established (35).

Based on the above background, the following research questions were proposed in the present study:

1. What are the perceptions of the program participants toward the Tier 2 program in the community-based P.A.T.H.S. Program? Previous results consistently revealed that the perceptions of the program participants were positive (25). Hence, we expected similar findings in this study (Hypothesis 1).
2. Are there any inter-relationships amongst the three aspects (program qualities, implementers qualities, and program effectiveness) assessed by Form C? Previous studies showed significant relationships among these three dimensions (36). Therefore, we also expected significant relationships among these dimensions (Hypotheses 2a, 2b and 2c).

3. Do perceived program quality and perceived implementer quality predict participants' views on the effectiveness of program? Based on previous findings (36), we hypothesized that these two qualities would predict perceived effectiveness of the program (Hypotheses 3a and 3b).

OUR STUDY

The participants of the current study were Secondary 1 to Secondary 3 students showing greater psychosocial needs. From 78 schools and 15 community centers, 4,245 participants took part in the Tier 2 Program of the Project P.A.T.H.S. in 2015. Among all of the participants, there were about 2,739 in Secondary 1, 1,848 in Secondary 2, and the rest 658 from Secondary 3.

To examine the participants' perception of the program, the Research Team developed a detailed and clear manual including the procedures and instructions for students to complete the evaluation form (Form C). An e-learning platform documenting all the procedures and instructions was also designed for collecting evaluation data using Form C. Once the program finished, the Form C was given to the students to complete. In the present study, a total of 3,958 completed questionnaires were collected.

Instruments

Comprising both rating scales and open-ended questions, the present study adopted a subjective outcome evaluation form (Form C) in the Tier 2 Program. Focus on understanding participants‘ perceptions, several major aspects including program content, implementer performance and program effectiveness were examined in Form C. For the structured assessment items, the present study used a 6-point scale (1 = "strongly disagree"; 6 = "strongly agree").

Data analyses

Descriptive statistics were used to examine the percentages of students' perceptions of the three dimensions of program ("program qualities", "implementer qualities," and "program effectiveness") in Form C. Reliability analysis was conducted to investigate the internal consistency of the scale. Pearson correlation analyses were performed to examine the inter-relationships amongst the three dimensions. Finally, multiple regression analyses were used to find whether the program and implementers qualities could predict the effectiveness of the program.

FINDINGS

Using descriptive data analysis, the current study examined the percentages of responses towards program qualities, implementer qualities, and program effectiveness based on Form C. Results revealed that great majority of the students held positive attitudes toward the program. Results in Table 1 showed that overall 95.4% respondents were satisfied with the program and perceived that "the activities were carefully planned" (95.3%). Approximately 94.8% of the respondents gave high recognition for the program. In Table 2, the same positive findings could be found regarding the participants' perceptions of the implementers. About 95.9% participants were satisfied with the workers and perceived that they had professional knowledge and well prepared for the program. Views toward program effectiveness also showed positive results (see Table 3): 94.2% of the respondents felt that the program was beneficial to their problem solving ability; 94% of them believed that the program could help their development.

Reliability analyses (see Table 4) showed that program content ($\alpha = .96$), program implementers ($\alpha = .96$), and program effectiveness ($\alpha = .96$) subscales as well as the total scale of Form C were reliable ($\alpha = .97$). Regarding the inter-relationships among the items on "program content"

(8 items), "program implementers" (8 items) and "program effectiveness" (8 items), Pearson correlation analyses (see Table 5) showed correlation between "program content" and "program effectiveness" ($r = .65$, $p < .001$), "program implementers" and "program effectiveness" ($r =.65$, $p < .001$), and "program content" and "program implementers" ($r = .77$, $p < .001$) in different grades.

Table 1. Comparison of the Positive Views towards Tier 2 Program across Different Grades

	Participants with positive responses across different grades							
	S1		S2		S3		Overall	
	N	%	N	%	N	%	N	%
The activities were carefully planned.	2396	94.9	803	95.9	573	96.3	3772	95.3
The quality of the service was high.	2385	94.4	795	95.0	571	96.0	3751	94.8
The service provided could meet the participants' needs.	2390	94.6	783	93.5	569	95.6	3742	94.5
The service delivered could achieve the planned objectives.	2385	94.4	791	94.5	567	95.3	3743	94.6
I could get the service I wanted.	2361	93.5	793	94.7	569	95.6	3723	94.1
I had much interaction with other participants.	2375	94.0	796	95.1	570	95.8	3741	94.5
I would recommend others who have similar needs to participate in the program.	2329	92.2	786	93.9	570	95.8	3685	93.1
On the whole, I am satisfied with the service.	2398	94.9	801	95.7	577	97.0	3776	95.4

Note: All items are on a 6-point Likert scale with 1 = strong disagree, 2 = disagree, 3 = slightly disagree, 4 = slightly agree, 5 = agree, 6 = strongly agree. Only respondents with positive responses (Options 4-6) are shown in the table.

Table 2. Comparison of the Positive Views towards Implementers of the Tier 2 Program across Different Grades

	Participants with positive responses across different grades							
	S1		S2		S3		Overall	
	N	%	N	%	N	%	N	%
The worker(s) has professional knowledge.	2408	95.3	811	96.9	575	96.6	3794	95.9
The worker(s) demonstrated good working skills.	2401	95.1	805	96.2	580	97.5	3786	95.7
The worker(s) was well prepared for the program.	2414	95.6	806	96.3	577	97.0	3797	95.9
The worker(s) understood the needs of the participants.	2396	94.9	797	95.2	574	96.5	3767	95.2
The worker(s) cared about the participants.	2407	95.3	805	96.2	573	96.3	3785	95.6
The worker(s)' attitudes were very good.	2403	95.1	806	96.3	581	97.6	3790	95.8
The worker(s) had much interaction with participants.	2360	93.4	800	95.6	574	96.5	3734	94.3
On the whole, I am satisfied with the worker(s).	2415	95.6	802	95.8	579	97.3	3796	95.9

Note: All items are on a 6-point Likert scale with 1 = strong disagree, 2 = disagree, 3 = slightly disagree, 4 = slightly agree, 5 = agree, 6 = strongly agree. Only respondents with positive responses (Options 4-6) are shown in the table.

Table 3. Comparison of the Positive Views towards the Effectiveness of the Tier 2 Program across Different Grades

	Participants with positive responses across different grades							
	S1		S2		S3		Overall	
	N	%	N	%	N	%	N	%
The service has helped me a lot.	2351	93.1	789	94.3	564	94.8	3704	93.6
The service has enhanced my growth.	2358	93.3	799	95.5	565	95.0	3722	94.0
In the future, I would receive similar service(s) if needed.	2323	92.0	780	93.2	570	95.8	3673	92.8
I have learned how to help myself through participating in the program.	2355	93.2	795	95.0	562	94.5	3712	93.8
I have had positive change(s) after joining the program.	2358	93.3	792	94.6	563	94.6	3713	93.8
I have learned how to solve their problems through participating in the program.	2368	93.7	793	94.7	568	95.5	3729	94.2
My behaviour has become better after joining this program.	2312	91.5	780	93.2	560	94.1	3652	92.3
Those who know me agree that this program has induced positive changes in me.	2306	91.3	788	94.1	561	94.3	3655	92.3

Note: All items are on a 6-point Likert scale with 1 = strong disagree, 2 = disagree, 3 = slightly disagree, 4 = slightly agree, 5 = agree, 6 = strongly agree. Only respondents with positive responses (Options 4-6) are shown in the table.

Table 4. Mean, standard deviations, Cronbach's alphas, and mean of inter-item correlations among the variables by grade

	S1		S2		S3		Overall	
	M (SD)	α (Mean#)	M (SD)	α (Mean#)	M (SD)	α (Mean#)	M (SD)	α (Mean#)
Program content (8 items)	4.98 (.83)	.96 (.73)	4.93 (.84)	.96 (.75)	4.99 (.78)	.96 (.75)	4.97 (.83)	.96 (.73)
Program implementers (8 items)	5.10 (.83)	.96 (.76)	5.10 (.83)	.97 (.79)	5.11 (.78)	.96 (.76)	5.10 (.82)	.96 (.77)
Program effectiveness (8 items)	4.94 (.87)	.96 (.74)	4.95 (.81)	.96 (.75)	5.01 (.77)	.96 (.73)	4.95 (.84)	.96 (.74)
Total effectiveness (24 items)	5.01 (.76)	.97 (.61)	4.99 (.70)	.97 (.55)	5.04 (.70)	.98 (.62)	5.01 (.74)	.97 (.60)

Mean inter-item correlations.

Table 5. Correlation coefficients on the relationship between program components and program effectiveness by grade

Variable	S1		S2		S3		Overall	
	1	2	1	2	1	2	1	2
1. Program content (8 items)	--		--		--		--	
2. Program implementers (8 items)	$.77^{***}$	--	$.73^{***}$	--	$.82^{***}$	--	$.77^{***}$	--
3. Program effectiveness (8 items)	$.69^{***}$	$.68^{***}$	$.53^{***}$	$.50^{***}$	$.65^{***}$	$.71^{***}$	$.65^{***}$	$.65^{***}$

$^{***}p < .001$.

Finally, multiple regression findings in Table 6 showed that program content (S1: $\beta = .41$, $p < .001$; S2: $\beta = .35$, $p < .001$; S3: $\beta = .21$, $p < .001$; Overall: $\beta = .38$, $p < .001$) and the program implementers (S1: $\beta = .36$, p <

.001; S2: β = .25, p < .001; S3: β = .53, p < .001; Overall: β = .35, p < .001) were significant predictors of program effectiveness.

Table 6. Multiple regression analyses predicting program effectiveness by grade

	Predictors			
	Program content	Program implementers	Model	
	β[a]	β[a]	R	R^2
S1	.41***	.36***	.73	.53
S2	.35***	.25***	.56	.31
S3	.21***	.53***	.72	.51
Overall	.38***	.35***	.69	.47

[a] Standardized coefficients.
****p* < .001.

DISCUSSION

Based on the data analyses of Form C collected from secondary school students with greater psychosocial needs, the present study was aimed to explore the effectiveness of the Tier 2 Program in the community-based phase of the P.A.T.H.S. Project in Hong Kong. As previous research suggested that PYD programs led to better outcomes for at-risk youth (37), it was expected that students joining the program would experience program benefits of the Tier 2 Program. There are several special features of the present study. First, this study used data collected from the community-based P.A.T.H.S. Project. The findings showed that the P.A.T.H.S. Tier 2 Program was equally effective in both school-based and community-based contexts. Second, the current study utilized the Form C that was found to have good psychometric properties (35). Third, a large sample size (N = 4,245) participated in this study. Fourth, in view of the lack of empirical research in the field of community-based PYD programs in the Chinese context, this study can be regarded as a pioneering attempt, which makes an important contribution to the Chinese literature on PYD programs.

With regard to the descriptive statistical analyses, several observations deserve attention. The current findings suggest that positive attitudes toward the Tier 2 program could be found in majority of students. Hence, Hypotheses 1 was supported. Specifically, more than 90% of the participants said that "they were satisfied with the service" and they highly recognized the program to be well-designed and implemented. Besides, positive attitudes could be found on the students' perceptions of program implementers and program effectiveness. In particular, an overwhelming majority of the students viewed that through joining the program, their problem solving skills as well as self-help skills improved. These benefits are of paramount importance for healthy youth development. For instance, previous research suggested that problem-solving abilities were negatively associated with the development of anxiety and depression (38). Problem-solving skills also prevented youth violence (39).

Consistent with previous studies, findings based on internal consistency and Pearson correlation analyses revealed that the Form C is valid and reliable. In particular, Pearson correlation analyses suggest that there were significant inter-correlations among the three dimensions (i.e., "program quality," "implementer quality," and "program effectiveness") across the three grade levels. The present findings are in line with the findings in previous studies (25, 31) and they provide support for Hypotheses 2a, 2b and 2c.

Considering the predictors of perceived program effectiveness, findings are consistent with our expectation. As both program content and program implementer quality were significant predictors of program effectiveness, findings are in line with the previous findings (36). Hence, Hypotheses 3a, and 3b were supported. With respect to program content in the community-based Tier 2 program, different program content based on the experiential learning approach was used to design different topic-related activities to help students strengthen their competence, cultivate their social responsibility, and promote prosocial behaviors. Besides, consistent with previous studies, quality of program implementers was also a significant predictor of participants' rating of program effectiveness. Thus, the current findings suggest that systematic training of program implementers, which would eventually shaping program quality, should be stepped up in positive youth development programs.

Several limitations of this research should be noted. First, as only quantitative subjective outcome evaluation findings were presented in this study, qualitative subjective outcome evaluation findings should be presented in future. Second, only findings based on the perceptions of the student participants were discussed. Hence, it would be interesting to include data based on the perspective of the program implementers as well. Third, in line with previous studies (25, 31), only perceptions of program content and implementer quality were considered as predictors in this study. This design may not be adequate and comprehensive enough. As such, other predictors such as parental involvement should be examined to explore their effect on program effectiveness in future research. Despite these limitations, the current findings provide further evidence suggesting that the community-based Tier 2 programs of the P.A.T.H.S. Project are effectiveness in promoting holistic development of adolescents with greater psychosocial needs.

ACKNOWLEDGMENTS

The preparation for this paper and the Project P.A.T.H.S. were financially supported by The Hong Kong Jockey Club Charities Trust. The materials in this chapter are based on a paper published in the *International Journal on Disability and Human Development* 2017;16 (4) issue.

REFERENCES

[1] Shek DTL, Hing KMA, Sun RCF. A brief overview of adolescent developmental problems in Hong Kong. ScientificWorldJournal 2011;11:2243-2256.

[2] Monahan KC. Adolescent pathways to co-occurring problem behavior: The effects of peer delinquency and peer substance use. J Res Adolescence 2014;24(4):630-45.

[3] Shek DTL, Yu L. Longitudinal impact of the Project P.A.T.H.S. on adolescent risk behavior: What happened after five years? ScientificWorldJournal 2012; 2012:316029.
[4] Book AS, Volk AA, Hosker A. Adolescent bullying and personality: An adaptive approach. Pers Individ Diff 2012;52(2):218-23.
[5] Wang J, Iannotti RJ, Nansel TR. School bullying among adolescents in the United States: Physical, verbal, relational, and cyber. J Adolesc Health 2009;45(4):368-75.
[6] Wang J, Iannotti RJ, Luk JW. Patterns of adolescent bullying behaviors: Physical, verbal, exclusion, rumor, and cyber. J Sch Psychol 2012;50(4):521-34.
[7] Mishna F. Risk factors for involvement in cyber bullying: Victims, bullies and bully–victims. Child Youth Serv Rev 2012;34(1):63-70.
[8] Cassidy W, Faucher C, Jackson M. Cyberbullying among youth: A comprehensive review of current international research and its implications and application to policy and practice. Sch Psychol Int 2013;34:575-612.
[9] Mackie CJ. Adolescent bullying, cannabis use and emerging psychotic experiences: A longitudinal general population study. Psychol Med 2013;43(5):1033-44.
[10] Foshee VA. Bullying as a longitudinal predictor of adolescent dating violence. J Adolesc Health 2014;55(3):439-44.
[11] Erignoz E. The role of parental, school, and peer factors in adolescent bullying involvement: Results from the Turkish HBSC 2005/2006 Study. Asia-Pacific J Public Health 2015;27(2):NP1591-603.
[12] Willford A. Effects of the KiVa anti-bullying program on adolescents' depression, anxiety, and perception of peers. J Abnorm Child Psychol 2012;40(2):289-300.
[13] Wang J, Nansel TR, Iannotti RJ. Cyber and traditional bullying: Differential association with depression. J Adolesc Health 2011;48(4):415-7.
[14] Ttofi MM, Farrington DP. Effectiveness of school-based programs to reduce bullying: A systematic and meta-analytic review. J Exp Criminology 2011;7(1):27-56.
[15] Swendsen J. Use and abuse of alcohol and illicit drugs in US adolescents: Results of the National Comorbidity Survey–Adolescent Supplement. Arch Gen Psychiatry 2012;69(4):390-8.
[16] Tanner-smith EE, Wilson SJ, Lipsey MW. The comparative effectiveness of outpatient treatment for adolescent substance abuse: A meta-analysis. J Subst Abuse Treat 2013;44(2):145-58.
[17] Narcotics Division. The 2014/15 Survey of Drug Use among Students. Hong Kong, Narcotics Division, Security Bureau, The Government of the Hong Kong, Special Administrative Region, 2015. URL: http://www.nd.gov.hk/en/survey_of_drug_use_14-15.htm.
[18] Shek DTL, Yu L. A review of validated youth prevention and positive youth development programmes in Asia. Int J Adolesc Med Health 2011;23:317-24.
[19] Damon W. What is positive youth development? Ann Am Acad Political Soc Sci 2004;591:13–24.

[20] Benson PL. Positive youth development: Theory, research, and applications. New York: John Wiley, 2006.

[21] Gavin LE. A review of positive youth development programs that promote adolescent sexual and reproductive health. J Adolesc Health 2010;46(3):75-91.

[22] Catalano RF. Prevention science and positive youth development: Competitive or cooperative frameworks? J Adolesc Health 2002;31(6):230-9.

[23] Catalano RF, Berglund ML, Ryan JAM, Lonczak HS, Hawkins JD. Positive youth development in the United States: Research findings on evaluations of positive youth development programs. Ann Am Acad Political Soc Sci 2004;591(1):98-124.

[24] Shek DTL, Yu L. A review of validated youth prevention and positive youth development programmes in Asia. Int J Adolesc Med Health 2011;23:317-24.

[25] Shek DTL, Sun RCF. Positive youth development programs for adolescents with greater psychosocial needs: Subjective outcome evaluation over 3 years. J Pediatr Adolesc Gynecol 2014;27:17-25.

[26] Shek DTL. Evaluation of the Project P.A.T.H.S. using multiple evaluation strategies. In: Development and evaluation of positive adolescent training through holistic social programs (P.A.T.H.S.). Singapore: Springer, 2013;53-67.

[27] Shek DTL, Sun RCF. Evaluation of positive youth development programs that help secondary 2 students with greater psychosocial needs. Int Public Health J 2009;1(3):335-46.

[28] Shek DTL, Hing KMA, Sun RCF. Development of a new curriculum in a positive youth development program: The Project P.A.T.H.S. in Hong Kong. ScientificWorldJournal 2011;11:2207-18.

[29] Kim BKE. Change in protective factors across adolescent development. J Appl Dev Psychol 2015;40:26-37.

[30] Walker JS, Gowen LK. Community-based approaches for supporting positive development in youth and young adults with serious mental health conditions. Research and Training Center for Pathways to Positive Futures. Portland, OR: Portland State University, 2011.

[31] Shek DTL, Ma CMS. Subjective outcome evaluation findings: Factors related to the perceived effectiveness of the Tier 2 Program of the Project P.A.T.H.S. ScientificWorldJournal 2010;10:250-60.

[32] Carpenter AT, Carpenter VG. Reflections of client satisfaction: Reframing family perceptions of mandatory alternative school assignment. J Instruct Psychol 2012;39:1-11.

[33] Shek DTL. Is subjective outcome evaluation related to objective outcome evaluation? Insights from a longitudinal study in Hong Kong. J Pediatr Adolesc Gynecol 2014;27:50-6.

[34] Shek DTL, Sun RCF. Secondary data analyses of subjective outcome evaluation findings of the Project P.A.T.H.S. in Hong Kong. ScientificWorldJournal 2010;10:2101-11.

[35] Shek DTL, Ma CMS, Siu AMH. Validation of a subjective outcome evaluation tool for participants in a positive youth development program in Hong Kong. J Pediatr Adolesc Gynecol 2014;27:26-31.

[36] Shek DTL, Law MYM. Evaluation of programs for adolescents with greater psychosocial needs: Community-based Project P.A.T.H.S. in Hong Kong. Int J Adolesc Med Health 2017;29(1):23-31.

[37] Sanders J, Munford R, Thimasarn-Anwar T. The role of positive youth development practices in building resilience and enhancing wellbeing for at-risk youth. Child Abuse Negl 2015;42:40-53.

[38] Hui EKP, Tsang SKM, Law BCM. Combating school bullying through developmental guidance for positive youth development and promoting harmonious school culture. ScientificWorldJournal 2012;5(1):2266-77.

[39] Wilson CJ, Bushnell JA, Rickwood DJ. The role of problem orientation and cognitive distortions in depression and anxiety interventions for young adults. Adv Ment Health 2011;10(1):52-61.

In: Soft Skills and Aspirations …
Editors: Daniel TL Shek, et al.
ISBN: 978-1-53614-092-7

Chapter 5

SUBJECTIVE OUTCOME EVALUATION OF THE COMMUNITY-BASED P.A.T.H.S PROJECT

Daniel TL Shek[1-5,*], PhD, FHKPS, BBS, SBS, JP, Janet TY Leung[1], PhD and Jing Wu[1], PhD

[1]Department of Applied Social Sciences,
The Hong Kong Polytechnic University, Hong Kong, PR China
[2]Centre for Innovative Programs for Adolescents and Families,
The Hong Kong Polytechnic University, Hong Kong, PR China
[3]Department of Social Work, East China Normal University,
Shanghai, PR China
[4]Kiang Wu Nursing College of Macau, Macau, PR China
[5]Division of Adolescent Medicine, Department of Pediatrics,
Kentucky Children's Hospital, University of Kentucky School of
Medicine, Lexington, Kentucky, US

ABSTRACT

The present chapter adopted subjective outcome evaluation to examine program effectiveness from the views of implementers (N=375) who

---

* Corresponding Author Email: daniel.shek@polyu.edu.hk.

implemented the community-based Tier 2 Program of the Project P.A.T.H.S. in Hong Kong. Results revealed that most of the program implementers were satisfied with the program content, their own performance, and program benefits. In agreement with previous studies, the satisfaction ratings of both program content and implementer performance positively predicted perceived program benefits. Regarding the influences of different program delivery approaches, programs with the "interest-enhancement" element received more positive evaluation from implementers than did the programs without that element. For programs with the "work-related" element, parental involvement significantly raised implementers' satisfaction ratings on their own performance. The current findings provided evidence for the effectiveness of the P.A.T.H.S. Tier 2 Program from the perspective of the implementers.

INTRODUCTION

Adolescence has been widely considered as a risky developmental period marked by the emergence and escalation of problematic behaviors, such as substance abuse, self-harm and suicide, and unhealthy lifestyles (1, 2). In Hong Kong, adolescent developmental issues such as mental health problems deserve public concern (3, 4). Shek (5) pointed out that for adolescents in Hong Kong nowadays, substance abuse, shop-lifting, mental health problems, underage sex, and youth unemployment are all growing problems. Besides, family and parenting problems are common issues in families with adolescent members (5). The prevalence of adolescent developmental issues is an alarm for the current and future society development of Hong Kong. Hence, there is an urgent need to prevent and reduce adolescent risk behavior.

Traditional problem-based adolescent prevention interventions were designed according to specific developmental problems. For example, the "Alcohol Treatment Targeting Adolescents in Need (ATTAIN)" Project was established to cognitively and behaviorally reduce alcohol and marijuana use among minority juvenile offenders in the US (6). However, there are many criticisms of such a "problem-based" approach. First, most of the problem-based interventions had unsatisfactory long-term effects (7, 8). Secondly, it is redundant and not practical to develop prevention programs for each specific adolescent developmental issue because of the correlated nature of problematic behaviors (5). Lastly, over-emphasis on adolescent "problems" and "weaknesses" may stigmatize adolescents.

In the past several decades, the strengths-based approach has emerged to overcome the shortcomings of the traditional paradigm (9). Martin Seligman stated that "Psychology is not just the study of weakness and damage; it is also the study of strength and virtue. Treatment is not just fixing what is broken; it is nurturing what is best within ourselves" (10, p.4). The strength-based approach emphasizes integrated youth development from an ecological perspective. It is argued that young people would be less likely to engage in risk behaviors if they acquire psychosocial competencies (11). With specific reference to the Hong Kong context, the Project "P.A.T.H.S. (Positive Adolescent Training through Holistic Social Programmes)" that has been launched since the 2005/2006 school year is a good example of the positive youth development approach.

Funded by the Hong Kong Jockey Club Charities Trust (HKJCCT), the P.A.T.H.S. Project was initiated with the collaboration of the Education Bureau, Social Welfare Department, and a research team comprising academics from five universities in Hong Kong. The P.A.T.H.S. Project has received overwhelmingly positive feedbacks during its first-stage of implementation (12, 13). Different stakeholders held positive views of the effectiveness of the program. Hence, the project was extended for another cycle for the participating schools to consolidate the implementation experience. Therefore, till the 2011/2012 school year, the project had been implemented on the basis of school contexts for seven years. To draw an all-around picture of the P.A.T.H.S. Project, process evaluation and outcome evaluation are the two basic forms used to evaluate the effectiveness of the programs. Given that the implementation process refers to program adherence, program receiver's engagement, goal attainment, and process-outcome linkage (14, 15), process evaluation methods including interim evaluation (16) and systematic management information collection based on a co-walker scheme (17) were adopted in evaluating P.A.T.H.S. Project. On the other hand, objective and subjective outcome evaluation methods were employed to focus on answering questions like whether or not the intended program goals and objectives have been met, as well as whether or not the program is effective and efficient (18). The existing evaluation studies have verified the success of the school-based programs by revealing high implementation quality, less problematic behaviors and enhanced positive psychosocial constructs in student participants, and high satisfaction ratings from different stakeholders (19-21).

However, researchers have found that clinical and community-based programs are more effective in changing specific behaviors than school-based programs (22). For example, Franklin and Corcoran reviewed the programs and practices for preventing adolescent pregnancy (23). They found that community-based programs (such as family planning clinics and girls clubs) were more efficient in reducing the pregnancy rates than school-based programs. Therefore, to further promote the P.A.T.H.S. Project in the community context, the third phase of the project implementation was formally started in 2013. During the third phase of implementation, community-based youth enhancement programs were developed and implemented by social workers in non-governmental organizations (NGOs), who also collaborated with school teachers (24). In the first two years of community-based program implementation, existing studies showed that the community-based P.A.T.H.S. Project was as effective as the school-based ones (25-28). Therefore, the present study attempted to replicate these findings in the third year implementation of community-based P.A.T.H.S. Project and to find out the factors influencing the effectiveness of the programs.

Two tiers of programs are included in the P.A.T.H.S. Project targeting different types of adolescents. The Tier 1 Program is a curricula-based program attempting to promote the development of all junior secondary school students in Hong Kong. On the other hand, Tier 2 Program targets students with greater psychosocial needs in behavioral, emotional, or social domains that take up nearly one-fifth of the population (19). Adopting the subjective outcome evaluation method, the present study focused on the effectiveness of the Tier 2 Program implemented in the year 2015.

One of the important features of outcome evaluation is that it could assess the perceptions and satisfaction levels of various important stakeholders (29). There is a consensus in the evaluation literature about the importance of involving views of multiple stakeholders, such as program receivers, program implementers, evaluators, and parents if the receivers are children (30-32). However, there is a research gap that most empirical studies have been devoted to understanding the program participants' views and neglected views of other stakeholders (33). There are several justifications for including the views of implementers in the Tier 2 Program. First, data based on different stakeholders tend to be more objective because it could achieve triangulation and avoid single-rater bias (34). Secondly, amongst all stakeholders, program implementers have the most first-hand information about how the program had been delivered, how the receivers reacted, and how the implementers themselves performed (35). Thirdly, evaluating program quality based on the implementers' perspective shows respect to the frontline professionals and provides them opportunities to have self-reflection (33). Therefore, implementers' perceptions of the Tier 2 Program would be evaluated in the current study.

To find out the factors influencing the effectiveness of the Tier 2 Program, two important aspects would be considered in the present study. First, while different approaches can be used in implementing Tier 2 Program, four types of approaches are most commonly employed. These included: a) adventure-based counseling approach (ABC); b) volunteer training and service such as volunteerism (VTS); c) work-related approach such as visiting workplaces and skills development (WORK); and d) interest-enhancement approach such as flower arrangement learning course (INT). A combination of two or more types of approaches is also common in implementing the Tier 2 Program.

The adventure-based counseling (ABC) and volunteer training and service (VTC) approaches were both developed on the basis of experiential learning theory. "Adventure-based counseling" is an experiential counseling technique that focuses on adolescents' group cooperation and interpersonal skills (36, 37). Activities adopting the ABC element help increase student participants' self-esteem and strengthen their social maturity in a group-counseling environment (38-40). "Volunteer training and service" activities also have positive influences on adolescents' social development (41).

Stressing on a "non-obligated" helping (42), volunteerism is conducive to promoting prosocial attitudes and reducing problematic behaviors in adolescents (43). Previous studies have consistently revealed the benefits of these two approaches (20, 21). Shek, Yu, and Ho (20) compared participants' ratings of the programs with different delivery modes and found that programs incorporating both ABC and VTS elements were more effective than programs incorporating solely ABC, solely VTS, or other delivery approaches (25). However, "work-related" and "interest-enhancement" activities also benefit adolescents' development practically. As for the importance of "work-related" element, Whiston and Quinby (44) reviewed several school counseling programs and concluded that career-related programs effectively promoted students' vocational identity, self-understanding, and the skills of connecting abilities with career choices. Regarding the "interest-enhancement" element, empirical studies showed that engaging in constructive extracurricular activities such as basketball or marching band promoted adolescents' school achievement and decreased their risky behaviors in the long run (45). Hence, interest enhancement activities are able to trigger the intrinsic motivation of the adolescents as a motivational strategy (46). Very few studies were concerned about the importance and effectiveness of the "WORK" and "INT" delivery approaches in the past. Accordingly, in the present study, WORK and INT in addition to VTS and ABC were taken into consideration to explore the effectiveness of different delivery approaches.

Apart from diverse approaches, the community-based Tier 2 programs were also different amongst themselves with respect to parental involvement. For some programs, only students with greater psychosocial needs participated in the activities. However, in some other programs, parent(s) were also involved. Some past studies have examined the effect of parental involvement and home-school relationship on adolescents' academic performance (e.g., 47, 48). Effective parental involvement in students' education not only strengthens children and adolescents' academic achievement and self-regulatory skills (49) but also promotes teachers' teaching efficacy and parents' own personal efficacy (50). However, possible barriers to the cooperation between parents and teachers also exist.

For parents, they may have inadequate skills without proper instructions. For teachers, they have to face the uncertainty when dealing with diverse families (48). Although the importance of parental involvement in adolescents' education has been well acknowledged, the effectiveness of parental involvement in positive youth development programs has seldom been considered in previous studies. Hence, the current study would try to fill this research gap.

Based on the aforementioned background, the present study evaluated the effectiveness of the Tier 2 Program of P.A.T.H.S. Project in Hong Kong in the 2015 year based on the program implementers' views. Several research questions to be addressed and hypotheses to be examined in the present study are listed as follows.

1) How satisfied were the program implementers regarding the program content, their performance, and program benefits? Since the previous studies steadily demonstrated positive feedback from the program implementers (21, 28), we hypothesized that program implementers would have a positive evaluation of the program content (Hypothesis 1a), implementer performance (Hypothesis 1b), and program benefits (Hypothesis 1c).
2) What are the inter-relationships amongst the ratings of program content, implementer quality, and program benefits? Based on previous findings, it was hypothesized that satisfaction ratings of the three aspects would be significantly associated with each other (Hypotheses 2a, 2b, and 2c). Furthermore, we hypothesized that satisfaction ratings of program content (Hypotheses 2d) and implementer quality (Hypotheses 2e) would both significantly predict that of program effectiveness.
3) Do grade differences exist when the program implementers appraise the program content, implementer quality, and program benefits? Grade differences were found in the Tier 1 Program from the perspective of implementers (e.g., 24), with lower grade teachers perceived higher program effectiveness and their own performance than did higher-grade teachers. However, grade differences among

implementers in the Tier 2 Program were seldom found (27, 28). Hence, using the findings based on the Tier 1 Program, we expected there would be grade differences (Hypothesis 3).

4) How would different delivery modes affect implementers' satisfaction ratings of the programs? Based on the findings of previous studies (28), we hypothesized that the ABC/VTS/WORK/INT elements would have positive influences on the effectiveness of the programs (Hypothesis 4).
5) How would parental involvement influence implementers' perceived program effectiveness? A few previous studies have implied the positive impacts of involving teachers or parents (47, 48). Based on these findings, we hypothesized that programs involving parent(s) would receive a more positive evaluation from the implementers than did programs not involving parent(s) (Hypothesis 5).

OUR STUDY

To understand the perceptions of implementers towards the program, researchers from the Project P.A.T.H.S. invited the implementers to complete a Subjective Outcome Evaluation Form for Instructors (Form D). It is a self-administrated questionnaire with clear guidelines and instructions. In the third year of implementation, we received 375 completed questionnaires, with 9 questionnaires with unclear information on the grade of the students.

Instruments

The Subjective Outcome Evaluation Form for Implementers (Form D) was employed at the end of the program. This measure covers three parts, which include a) instructors' views towards the program; b) instructors' views towards themselves; and c) instructors' perceived benefits of the program on the participants. Moreover, to collect additional comments from implementers, another four open-ended questions were also used to understand "a) important thing(s) the instructors have learned in the program; b) thing(s) that the instructors appreciate the most in the program; c) difficulties the instructors encountered; and d) areas of the program that need to be improved." In the present study, only the structured items were analyzed and reported. All structured items were assessed with items on a 6-point scale (from "strongly disagree" to "strongly agree").

Besides, additional information about the program was collected from the program implementers. Research assistants assisted to categorize the program delivery approaches according to the activities the NGOs conducted. On the other hand, types and numbers of participants for every program were also collected.

Data analyses

The basic units of analysis were individual data of the implementers in the current study. The SPSS 23.0 was used to generate all statistical analyses. First, the characteristics of the Tier 2 Program (delivery approach and types of participants) were categorized. Then, percentages of responses of the implementers regarding their views of the program (i.e., program qualities, program implementer qualities, and program benefits) were analyzed by descriptive statistics to test Hypotheses 1a to 1c. Moreover, the relationships among the above three areas were examined by Pearson correlation and multiple regression analyses to test Hypotheses 2a to 2e. To explore grade differences of implementers' subjective outcome evaluation (Hypothesis 3), a multivariate analysis of variance (MANOVA) was conducted using the evaluation of three aspects (i.e., program content, implementer performance, and program benefits) as dependent variables.

To investigate the influences of different delivery approaches and parental involvement on perceived program effectiveness, we first recoded the program approaches into four dichotomous variables for data analysis. For each of the four program approach variable (i.e., ABC, VTS, WORK, and INT), if the corresponding element was adopted in the program the variable was coded as "1," otherwise, it was coded as "0." Almost all programs adopted a combination of two or more elements. Likewise, the "parental involvement" variable was also coded according to the types of participants. Specifically, programs included parent(s) in the activities were coded as "1" for the "parental involvement" variable, while those without parental involvement coded as "0." To test Hypotheses 4 and 5, a series of ANOVA analyses were also performed with the three subjective outcome evaluation aspects (i.e., program content, implementers, and benefits) as dependent variables, and the four program approaches (ABC, VTS, WORK, and INT) as well as parental involvement as independent variables.

FINDINGS

In the year 2015, a total of 21 NGOs conducted 41 projects of the P.A.T.H.S. Tier 2 Programs. Most of the projects adopted more than one delivery approach. For example, twenty-two projects (N= 189) adopted the "ABC," "VTS," and "INT" elements at the same time, while 8 projects (N = 59) combined the four elements simultaneously. As demonstrated in Table 1, among all, the "adventure-based counseling" (ABC) element was the most frequently used (n=40), followed by the "volunteer training and service" (VTS) (n=39) and "interest-enhancement" (INT) (n=32) elements. The "work related" (WORK) element was also adopted by several projects (n=11). Besides the commonly adopted four approaches, parent(s) were actively involved in 12 projects.

As shown in Table 2, all of the three rating scales showed good internal consistency (α = .89 to .91). The Cronbach's alpha coefficient of the overall scale was .94, suggesting that the scales are reliable.

Table 1. Summary of the characteristics and effectiveness of the Tier 2 programs

Program Approach[1]	Parental Involvement	Average No. of Student participants	Average No. of Parent participants	Average No. of Teacher participants	Average Program Attendance (%)	Mean of Overall Effectiveness (M, SD)
ABC	Yes (*n*=12, *N*=95)	129.8	31.23	11.9	87.75	(5.07, .35)
	No (*n*=30, *N*=260)	88.0	N/A	8.3	84.62	(4.99, .40)
	Total (*n*=40, *N*=355)	99.3	8.44	9.3	85.46	(5.01, .39)
VTS	Yes (*n*=11, *N*=92)	131.71	31.76	12.1	87.81	(5.07, .35)
	No (*n*=29, *N*=250)	86.11	.00	7.8	84.48	(4.98, .42)
	Total (*n*=39, *N*=342)	98.60	8.70	9.0	85.39	(5.01, .40)
WORK	Yes (*n*=3, *N*=21)	98.3	15.55	14.3	85.90	(5.33, .33)
	No (*n*=8, *N*=58)	90.4	.00	6.7	88.06	(4.95, .44)
	Total (*n*=11, *N*=79)	92.5	4.15	8.7	87.48	(5.05, .45)
INT	Yes (*n*=8, *N*=54)	125.5	24.9	11.8	87.53	(5.17, .34)
	No (*n*=26, *N*=222)	87.4	.00	7.5	84.16	(5.00, .41)
	Total (*n*=32, *N*=276)	94.9	4.9	8.3	84.82	(5.03, .40)
Total	Yes (*n*=12, *N*=95)	128.9	31.0	11.8	87.72	(5.07, .35)
	No (*n*=31, *N*=280)	84.3	.00	8.0	84.89	(4.99, .42)
	Total (*n*=41, *N*=375)	95.6	7.9	9.0	85.61	(5.01, .40)

Notes: ABC= adventure-based counseling; VTS= volunteer training and service; WORK= work related; INT= interest-enhancement.

n= No. of projects; N= No. of implementers; N/A= not applicable.

[1] For each of the four program approach variable (i.e., ABC, VTS, WORK, and INT), if the corresponding element was adopted in the program the variable was coded as "1," otherwise, it was coded as "0." Almost all programs adopted a combination of two or more elements.

Table 2. Mean, standard deviations, Cronbach's alphas, and mean of inter-item correlations among the variables by grade

	Grade 7		Grade 8		Grade 9		Overall	
	M *(SD)*	*α* *(Mean)*	*M* *(SD)*	*α* *(Mean)*	*M* *(SD)*	*α* *(Mean)*	*M* *(SD)*	*α* *(Mean)*
Program content (8 items)	5.07 (.40)	.88 (.49)	5.01 (.47)	.89 (.50)	5.08 (.50)	.90 (.53)	5.07 (.44)	.89 (.51)
Program implementers (8 items)	5.04 (.44)	.89 (.52)	5.12 (.47)	.92 (.58)	5.10 (.45)	.89 (.49)	5.09 (.45)	.90 (.53)
Program benefits (8 items)	4.85 (.51)	.91 (.55)	4.86 (.52)	.91 (.55)	4.93 (.58)	.90 (.54)	4.88 (.53)	.91 (.55)
Total effectiveness (24 items)	4.98 (.38)	.94 (.39)	4.99 (.40)	.94 (.38)	5.01 (.43)	.94 (.40)	5.01 (.40)	.94 (.40)

Mean: inter-item correlations

Results of the descriptive data analysis showed that the program implementers were highly satisfied with the program content (see Table 3). Almost all implementers agreed that "the quality of the service was high" (99.2%) and "on the whole, I am satisfied with the service I conducted" (99.5%). Almost all (99.7%) of the implementers "would recommend others who have similar needs to participate in this program."

As demonstrated in Table 4, implementers were also very satisfied with their own performance in the activities. Nearly all implementers indicated that "my working skills were good" (99.7%) and "my attitudes were good" (99.7%). They were "satisfied with my performance on the whole" (99.7%). Furthermore, implementers believed that the Tier 2 programs had benefits for the participants (see Table 5). They indicated that the program "enhanced the participants to grow" (98.4%) and "participants have positive changes after joining the program" (98.1%). They also believed that in the future, "the participants would join similar programs if needed" (98.4%). Therefore, the Hypothesis 1a, 1b, and 1c in the present study were well supported

Table 3. Summary of the views of program implementers toward the program

	Implementers with positive responses (rating 4 to 6) across different grades							
	Grade 7		Grade 8		Grade 9		Overall	
	N	%	*N*	%	*N*	%	*N*	%
1) The activities were well planned.	207	98.1	87	100	68	100	371	98.9
2) The quality of the service was high.	208	98.6	87	100	68	100	372	99.2
3) The service provided could meet the participants' needs.	209	99.1	85	97.7	67	98.5	370	98.7
4) The service delivered could achieve the planned objectives.	208	98.6	85	97.7	66	97.1	368	98.1
5) I could provide the service participants wanted.	209	99.1	84	96.6	67	98.5	369	98.4
6) The program provided many chances for participants to interact with each other.	210	99.5	86	98.9	66	97.1	371	98.9
7) I would recommend others who have similar needs to participate in this program.	210	99.5	87	100	68	100	374	99.7
8) On the whole, I am satisfied with the service I conducted.	209	99.1	87	100	68	100	373	99.5

Note: All items are on a 6-point Likert scale with 1 = strongly disagree, 2 = disagree, 3 = slightly disagree, 4 = slightly agree, 5 = agree, 6 = strongly agree. Only respondents with positive responses (Options 4-6) are shown in the table.

regarding the associations among satisfaction ratings on program content, implementer quality, and program benefits, correlation analyses were conducted. As expected, significant positive correlations among program content, implementer quality, and perceived program benefits were found, with correlation coefficients ranging from .52 to .68 ($ps < .001$).

Table 4. Summary of the views of program implementers toward their own performance

	Implementers with positive responses (rating 4 to 6) across different grades							
	Grade 7		Grade 8		Grade 9		Overall	
	N	%	*N*	%	*N*	%	*N*	%
1) I used my professional knowledge.	209	99.1	87	100	68	100	373	99.5
2) My working skills were good.	210	99.5	87	100	68	100	374	99.7
3) I was well prepared for the program.	206	97.6	85	97.7	68	100	368	98.1
4) I understood the needs of the participants.	208	98.6	85	97.7	66	97.1	368	98.1
5) I cared about the participants.	209	99.1	87	100	68	100	373	99.5
6) My attitudes were good.	210	99.5	87	100	68	100	374	99.7
7) I had much interaction with participants.	208	98.6	87	100	67	98.5	371	98.9
8) On the whole, I am satisfied with my performance.	210	99.5	87	100	68	100	374	99.7

Note: All items are on a 6-point Likert scale with 1 = strongly disagree, 2 = disagree, 3 = slightly disagree, 4 = slightly agree, 5 = agree, 6 = strongly agree. Only respondents with positive responses (Options 4-6) are shown in the table.

Table 5. Summary of the program implementers' perceptions towards the benefits of the Tier 2 program

	Participants with positive responses (rating 4 to 6) across different grades							
	Grade 7		Grade 8		Grade 9		Overall	
	N	%	*N*	%	*N*	%	*N*	%
The program helped the participants a lot.	208	98.6	84	96.6	64	94.1	365	97.3
The program enhanced the participants to grow.	209	99.1	87	100	64	94.1	369	98.4
In the future, the participants would join similar program(s) if needed.	209	99.1	87	100	64	94.1	369	98.4
Participants have learnt how to help themselves through participating in the program.	208	98.6	85	97.7	63	92.6	365	97.3
Participants have positive change(s) after joining the program.	209	99.1	86	98.9	64	94.1	368	98.1

	Participants with positive responses (rating 4 to 6) across different grades							
	Grade 7		Grade 8		Grade 9		Overall	
	N	%	*N*	%	*N*	%	*N*	%
Participants have learned how to solve their own problems through participating in the program.	209	99.1	85	97.7	64	94.1	367	97.9
Compare with before joining this program, participants' behavior has become better.	205	97.2	84	96.6	61	89.7	359	95.7
Those who know the participants agree that this program has induced positive changes in them.	205	97.2	84	96.6	64	94.1	362	96.5

Note: All items are on a 6-point Likert scale with 1 = strongly disagree, 2 = disagree, 3 = slightly disagree, 4 = slightly agree, 5 = agree, 6 = strongly agree. Only respondents with positive responses (Options 4-6) are shown in the table.

The results supported Hypothesis 2a, 2b, and 2c. According to the results of multiple regression analyses, implementers' ratings on program effectiveness were significantly predicted by their satisfaction ratings on program content (β =.56, p <.001) and the ratings on their own performance (β =.21, p <.001). The positive inter-correlations and predictive relationships were also consistent across grades as indicated in Table 6 and Table 7. Therefore, Hypothesis 2d and Hypothesis 2e were also supported.

Table 6. Correlation coefficients on the relationship between program components and program benefits by grade

	Grade 7		Grade 8		Grade 9		Total	
Variables	2	3	2	3	2	3	2	3
1. Program content	.58***	.64***	.43***	.70***	.59***	.70***	.56***	.68***
2. Program implementers	-	.51***	-	.45***	-	.56***	-	.52***
3. Program benefits	-	-	-	-	-	-	-	-

***p < .001.

To explore the differences among implementers across grades when evaluating the program from three aspects, MANOVAs were conducted. According to the findings in Table 8, no significant grade differences were found among implementers when they were rating their satisfaction with program content (F (2,356)=.42, p =.66, η_p^2=.002), their own performance (F (2,356)=1.00, p =.37, η_p^2=.006), program benefits (F (2,356) = .54, p =.58, η_p^2=.003), as well as the overall program effectiveness (F (2,356) = .14, p =.87, η_p^2=.001). Hence, Hypothesis 3 that there would be grade differences among program implementers' satisfaction ratings was not supported in the present study.

Table 7. Multiple regression analyses predicting program benefits by grade

	Predictors			
	Program content	Program implementers	Model	
	β^a	β^a	R	R^2
Grade 7	.52***	.20**	.66	.43
Grade 8	.62***	.19*	.72	.52
Grade 9	.57***	.24*	.73	.54
Overall	.56***	.21***	.70	.49

a Standardized coefficients.

*p<.05; **p < .01; ***p < .001.

Table 8. Comparisons of the program evaluations by implementers in different grade levels

	***M* (*SD*)**			***df*1**	***df*2**	**MANOVA**	
	Grade 7 (N=207)	Grade 8 (N=87)	Grade 9 (N=65)			F	η_p^2
Program content	5.06(.40)	5.01(.47)	5.05(.50)	2	356	.42	.002
Program implementers	5.04(.44)	5.12(.47)	5.10(.45)	2	356	1.00	.006
Program benefits	4.85(.51)	4.86(.52)	4.93(.58)	2	356	.54	.003
Total effectiveness	4.98(.38)	4.99(.40)	5.01(.43)	2	356	.14	.001

To examine the impact of parental involvement and the delivery approaches, a series of ANOVAs were conducted with the three subjective outcome evaluation aspects (i.e., program content, implementer performance, and program benefits) as dependent variables, and the four program approaches (ABC, VTS, WORK, and INT) as well as parental involvement as independent variables.

Table 9. The impacts of parental involvement and delivery approaches on program effectiveness evaluated by implementers

Dependent Variables	Independent Variables	Yes		No		*F*	η_p^2
		N	*(M, SD)*	*N*	*(M, SD)*		
Program Content	*Main effects*						
	Parental involvement	94	5.12(.36)	274	5.04(.46)	1.53	.004
	ABC	348	5.08(.44)	20	4.96(.54)	1.36	.004
	VTS	336	5.07(.45)	32	5.05(.40)	.11	.000
	WORK	75	5.11(.48)	293	5.06(.43)	.20	.001
	INT	269	5.10(.47)	99	4.99(.43)	5.88*	.016
	Interaction effects[1]						
	Parental involvement* VTS					.07	.000
	Parental involvement* WORK					1.69	.005
	Parental involvement* INT					.98	.003
Program Implementers	*Main effects*						
	Parental involvement	94	5.14(.37)	274	5.06(.47)	2.54	.007
	ABC	348	5.09(.44)	20	5.06(.64)	.79	.002
	VTS	336	5.08(.45)	32	5.13(.47)	.68	.002
	WORK	75	5.13(.49)	293	5.07(.44)	.32	.001
	INT	269	5.11(.46)	99	5.00(.43)	7.71**	.021
	Interaction effects[1]						
	Parental involvement* VTS					.01	.000
	Parental involvement* WORK					7.67**	.021
	Parental involvement* INT					.36	.001
Program benefits	*Main effects*						
	Parental involvement	94	4.96(.45)	274	4.85(.55)	.86	.002
	ABC	348	4.88(.52)	20	4.89(.70)	.72	.002
	VTS	336	4.87(.53)	32	4.95(.53)	.27	.001
	WORK	75	4.98(.55)	293	4.86(.52)	2.35	.007
	INT	269	5.09(.53)	99	4.83(.51)	13.02***	.035
	Interaction effects[1]						
	Parental involvement* VTS					.10	.000
	Parental involvement* WORK					3.50	.010
	Parental involvement* INT					.50	.001

Notes: ABC= adventure-based counseling; VTS= volunteer training and service; WORK= work related; INT= interest-enhancement.

* $p < .05$; ** $p < .01$; *** $p < .001$.

[1] There are no interaction effects between parental involvement and the ABC approach since all programs that involved parent(s) adopted the ABC activities.

Table 10. Simple effect analysis of the interactions between "WORK" element and "parental involvement" on perceived implementer performance

		Parental Involvement				F	η_p^2
		Yes		No			
		N	(M, SD)	N	(M, SD)		
WORK	Yes	20	(5.42, .35)	55	(4.98, .47)	14.66***	.167
	No	74	(5.06, .34)	219	(5.08, .47)	.159	.001

Note: *** p < .001.

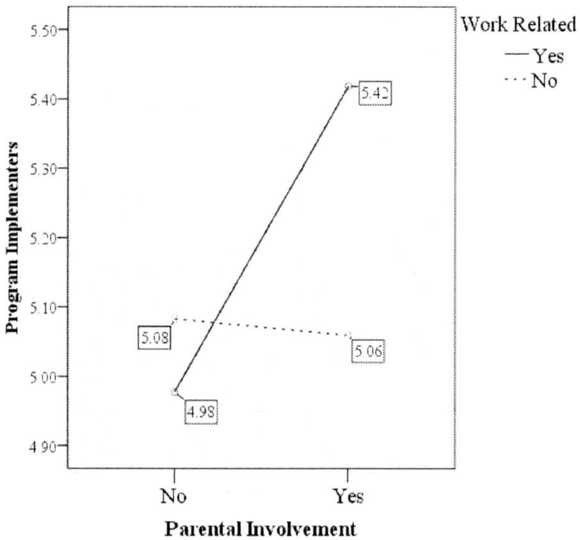

Figure 1. Simple effect analysis of the interactions between "WORK" element and "parental involvement" on perceived implementer performance.

DISCUSSION

Adolescents' problematic behaviors may result in academic failure, physical or psychological harms, and even social issues (1, 2). The Project P.A.T.H.S. is a strength-based youth development program that tailored to help adolescents in Hong Kong from an ecological perspective (5). This article examined the effectiveness of the community-based Tier 2 Program of the

Project P.A.T.H.S. implemented in the year 2015 from the views of 375 implementers.

According to the present findings based on subjective outcome evaluation, the program was successfully implemented as expected. It has received quite positive evaluation from the implementers in the aspects of perceived program content, self-perceived performance, and perceived program benefits. The overall perceived program effectiveness ranged from 3.46 to 6.00 on a six-point Likert scale. One of the big concerns when designing the community-based Tier 2 Program was whether it could be as effective as the school-based programs. The findings in the present study solidly supported the effectiveness of the community-based programs. It is delightful to observe the successful outcomes due to a valuable collaboration between social workers in NGOs and teachers in schools. Meanwhile, no grade differences were found in the subjective outcome evaluation results. The findings were in agreement with Shek, Ng, and Law's study (27). One possible explanation could be that Tier 2 programs conducted in three grades were equally effective and that implementers of all grades were equally satisfied with their own performance.

In line with the findings of previous studies (21, 27), the satisfaction ratings of both program content and implementer performance positively predicted perceived program benefits. The prediction effects were consistent across grades. These findings imply that in order to promote the holistic development of adolescents in different areas (such as emotional competence, prosocial norms, bonding, and self-efficacy), the program content should be well-designed and the implementers should be well-trained and wholehearted. Shek and colleagues (51) proposed that factors influencing the program quality could be concluded as 5 "P"s (policy, program, people, place, and process). The findings being presented echo the 5P model by identifying the importance of "program" and "people." In future studies, the other three factors could also be considered.

Different types of delivery approaches were used in the community-based Tier 2 Programs. Previous studies indicated that students had the highest preference for the adventure-based counseling (ABC) and volunteer training and service (VTC) approaches (25, 43). Owing to the successful implementation experience, almost every project incorporated the ABC and/or VTC element(s) during 2015. However, also due to the over-widened gap of the number of participants (355 implementers were in programs with the "adventure-based counselling" element while only 20 were not; 342 implementers were in programs with the "volunteer training and service" element while only 33 were not), the positive influence of adopting ABC and VTS approach on the program effectiveness was not successfully found in the present study. On the other hand, adopting "interest-enhancement" approach was found to have positive influences on implementers' satisfaction ratings in program content, implementer quality, and program benefits, which are new findings in evaluation studies for the P.A.T.H.S. Project. Interest-enhancement activities motivate adolescents to learn and practice with enthusiasm (46). In that way, implementers would also be activated and encouraged to make the activities more interesting and interactive. In the future, a further investigation of the impacts of the combination of different approaches should be considered.

Although no main effect was found to demonstrate the positive influence of parental involvement, the interaction effect between parental involvement and "work-related" element partially supported the benefits of parental involvement in youth development program. A previous study found that students preferred the programs involving only students more than the programs also involving parents (52). It is understandable that implementers valued the potential benefits for students more, while participated students preferred more relaxing experiences without parents' restrictions. Involving parents in "work-related" activities not only inspires parents to help kids' career development, but also contributes to the affectional ties within families. From the ecological perspective, supportive parents and teachers could provide protective factors for the adolescents at a community level (12).

Despite the above-mentioned contributions, the present study has several limitations. First, a fundamental concern for subjective outcome evaluation is the social desirability and self-serving bias because most of the responses were quite positive. It is human nature that individuals, including the program implementers, tend to perceive own performance as positive

(53). Therefore, a combination of both subjective and objective outcome evaluations from the perspectives of other stakeholders would be necessary. Second, since the community-based Tier 2 Program was mainly developed and implemented by NGO social workers, it would be difficult for research team members to master the details of the implementation process. Hence, qualitative evaluation measures, such as focus group and individual interviews, would be helpful to better evaluate and improve the programs. Third, a larger sample size would substantially enhance the generalizability of the findings in the current study. For example, the efficiency of parental involvement could not be well examined without sufficient participants. Future evaluating studies could also consider about their voices. Notwithstanding these limitations, the current study provided evidence for the success and effectiveness of the community-based Tier 2 Program of the P.A.T.H.S. Project. It also shed light on the future improvement of positive youth development programs.

Acknowledgments

The preparation for this paper and the Project P.A.T.H.S. were financially supported by The Hong Kong Jockey Club Charities Trust. The materials in this chapter are based on a paper published in the *International Journal on Disability and Human Development* 2017;16(4) issue.

References

[1] Omer H, Lebowitz ER. Nonviolent resistance: Helping caregivers reduce problematic behaviors in children and adolescents. J Marital Fam Ther, 2016;42(4):688-700.

[2] Donovan JE, Jessor R. Structure of problem behavior in adolescence and young adulthood. J Consult Clin Psychol 1985;53(6):890-904.

[3] Shek DTL. Adolescent developmental issues in Hong Kong: Relevance to positive youth development programs in Hong Kong. Int J Adolesc Med Health 2006;18 (3):341-54.

[4] Ho SMY, Lee TMC. Computer usage and its relationship with adolescent lifestyle in Hong Kong. J Adolesc Health 2001;29(4):258-66.
[5] Shek DTL, Ma HK, Sun RCF. A brief overview of adolescent developmental problems in Hong Kong. ScientificWorldJournal 2011;11:2243-56.
[6] Gil AG, Wagner EF, Tubman JG. Culturally sensitive substance abuse intervention for Hispanic and African American adolescents: Empirical examples from the Alcohol Treatment Targeting Adolescents in Need (ATTAIN) Project. Addiction 2004;99(s2):140-50.
[7] Botvin GJ, Baker E, Filazzola AD, Botvin EM. A cognitive-behavioral approach to substance abuse prevention: One-year follow-up. Addict Behav 1990;15(1):47-63.
[8] Sosin MR, Bruni M, Reidy M. Paths and impacts in the progressive independence model: A homelessness and substance abuse intervention in Chicago. J Addict Dis 1996;14(4):1-20.
[9] Smith EJ. The strength-based counseling model. Couns Psychol 2006;34(1):13-79.
[10] Martin S. Building resilience from the grassroots up. Monit Psychol 2002;33(11):52-3.
[11] Jessor R, Turbin MS, Costa FM, Dong Q, Zhang H, Wang C. Adolescent problem behavior in China and the United States: A cross-national study of psychosocial protective factors. J Res Adolesc 2003;13(3):329-60.
[12] Shek DTL, Leung JTY. Adolescent developmental issues in Hong Kong: Phenomena and implications for youth service. In: Shek DTL, Sun RCF, eds. Development and evaluation of positive adolescent training through holistic social programs (P.A.T.H.S.). Singapore: Springer, 2013:1-13.
[13] Shek DTL, Sun RCF. The Project PATHS in Hong Kong: Development, training, implementation, and evaluation. J Pediatr Adolesc Gynecol 2013;26(3):S2-9.
[14] Law BMF, Shek DTL. Process evaluation of a positive youth development program in Hong Kong based on different cohorts. ScientificWorldJournal 2012;2012:1-9.
[15] Scheirer MA. Designing and using process evaluation. Handb Pract Program Eval 1994;5:40-68.
[16] Shek DTL, Ma HK, Sun RCF. Interim evaluation of the Tier 1 Program (Secondary 1 Curriculum) of the Project PATHS: First year of the full implementation phase. ScientificWorldJournal 2008;8:47-60.
[17] Shek DTL, Sun RCF, Kan VW. Full implementation of the Secondary 1 program of Project PATHS: Observations based on the co-walker scheme. ScientificWorldJournal 2009;9:982-91.
[18] Schalock RL. Outcome-based evaluation. New York: Springer Science & Business Media, 2001.
[19] Shek DTL, Yu L. Subjective outcome evaluation of the Project PATHS (extension phase) based on the perspective of program implementer. ScientificWorldJournal 2012;2012:1-8.

[20] Shek DTL, Yu L, Ho VYT. Subjective outcome evaluation and factors related to perceived effectiveness of the Project PATHS in Hong Kong. ScientificWorldJournal 2012;2012:1-10.

[21] Shek DTL, Siu AMH, Lee TY. Subjective outcome evaluation of the Project PATHS: Findings based on the perspective of the program implementers. ScientificWorldJournal 2007;7:195-203.

[22] Hofferth SL. The effects of programs and policies on adolescent pregnancy and childbearing. In Hofferth SL, Hayes CD, eds. Risking the future: Adolescent sexuality, pregnancy and childbearing. Washington, DC: Department of Education, 1987:207-63.

[23] Franklin C, Corcoran J. Preventing adolescent pregnancy: A review of programs and practices. Soc Work 2000;45(1):40-52.

[24] Shek DTL, Wu FK. The Project PATHS in Hong Kong: Work done and lessons learned in a decade. J Pediatr Adolesc Gynecol 2016;29(1):S3-11.

[25] Shek DTL, Zhu XQ, Wu FK. Subjective outcome evaluation of the community-based program of the P.A.T.H.S. project in Hong Kong. Int J Child Adolesc Health 2017;10(2):139-51.

[26] Shek DTL, Law MYM. Evaluation of programs for adolescents with greater psychosocial needs: Community-based Project PATHS in Hong Kong. Int J Adolesc Med Health 2017;29(1):23-31.

[27] Shek DTL, Ng CSM, Law MYM. Positive youth development programs for adolescents with greater psychosocial needs: Evaluation based on program implementers. Int J Child Adolesc Health 2017;29(1):33-9.

[28] Shek DTL, Lin L. Project P.A.T.H.S. for adolescents with greater psychosocial needs: Evaluation based on the program implementers. Int J Child Adolesc Health 2017;10(2):153-63.

[29] Forman SG, Olin SS, Hoagwood KE, Crowe M, Saka N. Evidence-based interventions in schools: Developers' views of implementation barriers and facilitators. Sch Ment Health 2009;1(1):26-36.

[30] Taut S. What have we learned about stakeholder involvement in program evaluation? Stud Educ Eval 2008;34(4):224-30.

[31] Cousins JB, Whitmore E. Framing participatory evaluation. New Dir Eval 1998;1998(80):5-23.

[32] Greene JC. Stakeholder participation in evaluation design: Is it worth the effort? Eval Program Plann 1987;10(4):379-94.

[33] Sun RCF, Shek DTL. Perceived program qualities and outcomes of a youth program in Hong Kong based on the views of the workers. J Pediatr Adolesc Gynecol 2014;27:S10-6.

[34] House ER. Stakeholder bias. New Dir Eval 2003;2003(97):53-6.

[35] Winefield HR, Barlow, JA. Client and worker satisfaction in a child protection agency. Child Abuse Negl 1995;19(8):897-905.

[36] Glass JS, Shoffner MF. Adventure-based counseling in schools. Prof Sch Couns 2001;5(1):42-8.

[37] Moote GTJr, Wodarski JS. The acquistion of life skills through adventure-based activities and programs: A review of the literature. Adolescence 1997;32(125):143-67.

[38] Harris PM, Mealy L, Matthews H, Lucas R, Moczygemba M. A wilderness challenge program as correctional treatment. J Offender Rehabil 1993;19(3-4):149-64.

[39] Koperski H, Tucker AR, Lung DM, Gass MA. The impact of community based adventure therapy on stress and coping skills in adults. The Practitioner Scholar: J Couns Prof Psychol 2015;4(1):1-16.

[40] Hinduja S, Patchin JW. Cyberbullying: Neither an epidemic nor a rarity. Eur J Dev Psychol 2012;9(5):539-43.

[41] Penner LA. Volunteerism and social problems: Making things better or worse? J Soc Issues 2004;60(3):645-66.

[42] Omoto AM, Snyder M. Sustained helping without obligation: Motivation, longevity of service, and perceived attitude change among AIDS volunteers. J Pers Soc Psychol 1995;68(4):671-86.

[43] Allen JP, Kuperminc G, Philliber S, Herre K. Programmatic prevention of adolescent problem behaviors: The role of autonomy, relatedness, and volunteer service in the Teen Outreach Program. Am J Community Psychol 1994;22(5):595-615.

[44] Whiston SC, Quinby RF. Review of school counseling outcome research. Psychol Sch 2009;46(3):267-72.

[45] Eccles JS, Barber BL. Student council, volunteering, basketball, or marching band what kind of extracurricular involvement matters? J Adolesc Res 1999;14(1):10-43.

[46] Kobayashi M, Lockee B. Evidence-based approaches for self-regulated learning. Educ 2008;5:32-44.

[47] Epstein JL, Sanders MG. Prospects for change: Preparing educators for school, family, and community partnerships. Peabody J Educ 2006;81(2):81-120.

[48] Hoover-Dempsey KV, Walker JMT, Jones KP, Reed RP. Teachers Involving Parents (TIP): Results of an in-service teacher education program for enhancing parental involvement. Teach Teach Educ 2002;18(7):843-67.

[49] Zellman GL, Waterman JM. Understanding the impact of parent school involvement on children's educational outcomes. J Educ Res 1998;91(6):370-80.

[50] Hoover-Dempsey KV, Sandler HM. Parental involvement in children's education: Why does it make a difference? Teach Coll Rec 1995;97(2):310-31.

[51] Shek DTL, Sun RCF. Implementation of a positive youth development program in a Chinese context: The role of policy, program, people, process, and place. ScientificWorldJournal 2008;8:980-96.

[52] Shek DTL, Tsui PF, Law MYM. Evaluation of a school-based positive youth development program in Hong Kong: Views of junior secondary school students. Int J Child Health Hum Dev 2015;8(2):167-79.

[53] Miller DT, Ross M. Self-serving biases in the attribution of causality: Fact or fiction? Psychol Bull 1975;82(2):213-25.

SECTION TWO: DREAMS

In: Soft Skills and Aspirations … ISBN: 978-1-53614-092-7
Editors: Daniel TL Shek, et al.

Chapter 6

DREAMS AND ASPIRATIONS FOR LIFE

Daniel TL Shek[1-5,*], PhD, FHKPS, BBS, SBS, JP,
Florence KY Wu[1], BA, MASGC, EdD
and Hildie Leung[1], PhD
[1]Department of Applied Social Sciences,
The Hong Kong Polytechnic University, Hong Kong, PR China
[2]Centre for Innovative Programmes for Adolescents and Families,
The Hong Kong Polytechnic University, Hong Kong, PR China
[3]Department of Social Work, East China Normal University,
Shanghai, PR China
[4]Kiang Wu Nursing College of Macau, Macau, PR China
[5]Division of Adolescent Medicine, Kentucky Children's Hospital,
University of Kentucky, Lexington, Kentucky, US

ABSTRACT

Although children and adolescents are often asked about their "dreams" about life, scientific studies of "dreams" and related constructs are grossly inadequate. This chapter describes the findings arising from a review study exploring the concepts of dreams, aspirations and related constructs in

[*] Corresponding Author Email: daniel.shek@polyu.edu.hk.

children and adolescents. Besides an overview of the concept of dream, conceptual features and unique underpinnings of other concepts commonly related to dream, such as "aspirations," "hope," "future orientation" and "resilience" are examined in this chapter. The research questions surrounding "dream" and related constructs in children and adolescents are presented and future research directions are discussed.

INTRODUCTION

It is common for adults to ask children and adolescents what dreams they have. In primary and secondary schools, students are usually asked to write essays about their dreams and aspirations of life. However, when we asked whether the dreams of children and adolescents have been scientifically studied, two observations emerged. First, except the psychoanalytic literature on dreams, where dreams are regarded as the "royal road to the unconsciousness," systematic investigation of dreams in children and adolescents is sparse in the scientific literature. Second, dreams in children and adolescents are not necessarily described in a positive manner, particularly in the Chinese culture. Students who do not concentrate during class are labeled as "daydreamers." Young people who think big are also regarded as dreaming the impossible.

While few systematic research on the dreams of children and adolescents have been conducted, some related concepts such as aspirations, beliefs in the future and hope have been published. Benson (1) argued that developmental assets are "building blocks of healthy development that are essential for all youth, regardless of their background" (1). For example, one of the developmental assets conducive for positive youth development is beliefs in the future, including the development of future potentials, choices, goals, and options (2). Particularly, Sun and Shek (3) asserted that "promotion of beliefs in the future for positive youth development deserves greater attention since there is growing research evidence demonstrating its positive effects on adolescent well-being" (3). They recommended the provision of a supportive environment to encourage adolescents to internalize both hope and optimism. Against this background, there is a need to systematically review the scientific literature on dreams and the related constructs such as aspirations, hope, resilience, belief in the future and future orientation of children and adolescents to understand what factors shape their formation and how they affect adolescent development.

With the financial support of the Bao Bao Bear Care Foundation Limited, a collaborative research was conducted to understand the scientific underpinnings of instilling dreams, aspirations, hope, future orientation and related qualities in children and adolescents. The study attempted to investigate the positive impact of such constructs on children's and adolescents' well-being and overall development, as well as to review existing interventions based on the related constructs (4). The Bao Bao Care Foundation was founded in 2008 following the Sichuan earthquake to facilitate the provision of programs to children in Sichuan. As children should not be deprived of experiencing a sense of hope despite adversity, the iDream initiative was established to inspire and encourage children to explore their dreams, and to help ensure their positive future orientation. With an emphasis of exposing the children to the success stories of various professionals, it is believed that children would be able to understand the life trajectory leading to success and generate hope for their own future.

Based on the final report (4), three papers are included in the present special issue. In this paper, the basic concept of dream and the related constructs such as aspirations, and future orientation are discussed. The questions surrounding these concepts and the related observations are presented. Finally, the conclusions based on the literature review are highlighted. In the second paper, the methodology of the review and factors influencing dreams and related development are presented. The last paper discusses the existing interventions, instruments and consequences of these constructs on child developmental outcomes.

DREAMS AND THE RELATED CONSTRUCTS

Walt Disney once said that "if you can dream it, you can do it." Disney's quote attempted to state the causal relationship between "dream" (the manifestation of beliefs in the future) and "do" (action-taking to actualize the "dreams"). However, the manifestation of these beliefs depends on "*can*" -- an individual's ability to understand the unique meanings of "dream" to himself or herself, and the courage to create his/her own dream(s). Children and adolescents have often been claimed as "big dreamers." Yet the increasing trend of children and adolescents being despaired and hopeless hinders their boldness to "dream for future" and threatens their holistic well-being and health (5). Many educators, psychologists or professionals in human services have placed an increasing emphasis on how to nurture hope for the future in children and adolescents so that it helps to foster healthy development (6). However, in both Western and Chinese contexts, there is limited research on intervention programs assisting the children and adolescents to explore the meaning of "dream" uniquely to them.

Although there is scarce research about "dream" with reference to future hope, there has been a bloom of research on related concepts to "dream," namely "hope," "aspirations," "future orientation," "resilience" and "beliefs in the future." It is therefore fundamental to explore the meanings of "dream" and the related concepts (hope, aspirations, future orientation, resilience, and beliefs in the future) to children and adolescents, factors leading to the development of and possible outcomes of having developed these attributes in youth, and effective interventions implemented to help youngsters nurture these hope and aspirations in their life experiences. In this paper, we first outline the concepts in the literature review.

Dreams

"Dreams" are a specialized area of psychoanalytic research in Psychology. Freud, an advocator of researching dreams, stated that the functions of the dreams "as the guardians of sleep" have two distinctive characteristics – "wish-fulfillment and hallucinatory experience" (7). The notion falls much onto the psychological-neurobiological perspective in understanding what "dream" is. There is scarce literature reviewing the concept of "dream" apart from this framework. However, the idea "dream" in recent research of hopes or aspirations sheds lights upon some new interpretations of the concept. "Dream" appears to mean an individual's "wish" for the future and shares certain commonalities with the concepts of "hope" or "beliefs in the future" to manifest an individual's goals or beliefs at present (5, 8). In the study of Juvakka and Kylmä (5), the researchers investigated the meaning of hope in adolescents with cancer and the concept "dream" was often brought up by adolescent patients. The adolescents expressed their understanding of "dream" as "extended towards the future quite far away and they relate [dreams], for example, to studying and getting married and having children" or "being able to travel or having a boy or girlfriend" (p. 195). The "dreams" adolescents shared in the study were like Freudian explanation as "wish-fulfillment" yet no concrete plans or pathways were suggested (or not knowing how) to actualize these wishes. The wish to "study" and "establish a family" in their sharing, however, does engender hope in adolescents and exhibit their beliefs in the future.

"Dream" is "*meng-xiang*" in Chinese and it comprises "wish" or "dream" ("*meng*") and "thinking" ("*xiang*"). The "xiang" could be the imagined wishes ("*xiang-xiang*") or the cognitive process of actualizing the goals ("*li-xiang*"). In the Chinese context, no scientific study has been conducted to examine the concept of "dream" in adolescents. In Li's (9) action research, he assured the importance of pursuing children's own dreams in developing their moral values. The dreams to be pursued are "peer dreams" (the shared dream in adolescents), "great people dream" (the nurturance of leadership), "China dream" (the civic responsibility) and "world dream" (the contribution made to the world). Though each dream is not explicitly explained in this action research, the "dream" for Chinese children and adolescents is not limited to individual pursuit yet together with the cultural and national contexts.

Aspirations

In their conceptual review, Quaglia and Cobb (10) asserted that aspiration consists of two components: inspirations and future ambitions. "Inspiration" is experienced when an activity is perceived to be enjoyable and exciting. One is aware of being immersed in the here and now of life. "Ambitions" is characterized by the perception that a particular activity is meaningful toward the pursuance of a future goal. Based on the Social Cognitive Career Theory, Rojewski (11) suggested that self-efficacy beliefs and external socialization patterns including gender, socioeconomic status, and culture, as well as the internalization of learning experiences are important sources for aspirations. Thus, aspirations may be seen as inspiration served to motivate students toward their ambitions. Nurmi (12) explained the psychological processes of aspirations as motivation, planning, and evaluation. Motivation pertains to "what" future interests adolescents may have (i.e., goal-setting based on values and interests). Planning is about "how" one may achieve their prescribed goals (i.e., developing strategies). Evaluation is to do with assessing the possibility or extent that the goals may be actualized. Aspiration has long been perceived as a crucial psychological aspect of "a student's propensity towards post-secondary education and college attendance" and has been defined as the "educational and vocational dreams that students have for their future" (13). This notion emphasizes the role of aspiration in helping children and adolescents in achieving educational attainments and successes in their school and post-school years. Scholars have found that aspirations contribute significantly to educational and occupational achievements of children and adolescents (14, 15) and there are numerous studies investigating the relationship between academic outcomes and aspirations (13, 16, 17).

However, some scholars suggested that aspirations could be perceived from a developmental perspective and conceived them as future-oriented representations of what individuals strive for in various life domains (18). The meaning of the concepts "success" and "achievement" for children and adolescents is not only limited to academic attainments but also extended to other facets of life achievements. Aspirations or "career aspirations" may help elucidate on many important career development choices one makes across the lifespan (e.g., deciding on education pathways, making career-related choices) and how one perceives the availability of resources and the impact of social forces on one's career or life opportunities (11).

Hope

There are tremendous studies on the concept of "hope" in various professional arenas (e.g., psychology, theology, mental health or medical science). The theory of hope advocated by Snyder and his colleagues (19) has aroused much attention in recent literature. Snyder (20) defined hope as "a positive motivational state that is based on an interactively derived sense of successful agency (goal-directed energy) and pathways (planning to meet goals)" (20). The theory proposed by Snyder and his colleagues (19) gives equal emphasis on both the "agency" and "pathways" and states that an individual's hope level is not only depending on *how* one realizes his/her own goals ("pathways"), but also the one's *perceived ability* ("agency") to achieve those goals. This theory has influenced much of the recent research in conceptualizing hope to investigate if hope (one's agency and pathways) is relatively constant or hope levels fluctuate with a given situation (21).

Hope is conceptually distinct from other strength-based constructs like optimism (22) and self-efficacy (23). Although both hope and optimism focus on positive happenings in the future, optimism refers to the belief of "good rather than bad things will happen" (22) and hope puts this belief into action and generates plans for the future. Bailey et al. (24) explained this by noting that "[o]ptimism theory posits that outcome expectancies determine goal-directed behaviour, whereas hope theory posits that efficacy expectancies (agency) are equally necessary determinants of goal-directed behaviour."

Hope is a motivational construct found to be related to various positive outcomes in children, adolescents, and adults (25). High-hope children and adolescents have found to have an expectancy of success where the obstacles are perceived as "temporary," and the high level of goal-directed motivation allows impediment being channeled toward "the best alternative way" (26). Psychologists have found empirical evidence to support that hope is related to positive outcomes among youths including higher levels of goal-directed thinking (19), better use of coping strategies, as well as higher task performance (27, 28).

In spite of the attention to an individual motivation to sustain hope in life, little attention has been given to how the contextual assets help shape hope during childhood and adolescence (29). Te Riele (30) conceptualized hope in terms of four practical resources a) a focus on the possibility; b) a critical reflection of life's opportunity; c) a community of hope; and d) a positive culture for hope to thrive. These four resources affirm the interdependence of individual strength (an individual's perception of possibilities and reflections) and the ecology (the significant others and the culture) around the youth to nurture hope in children and adolescents. Yohani (8) observed that hope could be nurtured in the context of caring relationships from significant others. In addition, for children, caregivers' ability to devise ways for goal attainment is crucial to hope and adaptation (26). These caring and hopeful experiences of children and adolescents within their ecology are important predictors of hope during adolescence (31).

Factors engendering hope in children and adolescents are worth exploring with reference to their physical, psychological, or mental well-being and different cultural contexts. More research is warranted to better understand the conditions under which hope may operate and bring positive impact as a psychological strength. For instance, future studies may investigate the interactions between hope and different life experiences of children and adolescents (32).

Future orientation

According to Seginer et al. (33), future orientation is an umbrella term encapsulating different aspects of future thinking and the subjective image that one may have regarding a future time point. Future orientation relates much to the concepts "hope" and "aspiration." It is not to be mistaken with the prediction of the future, but rather, what one hopes for (or wishes not to happen) in the future. Future orientation is a complex and multidimensional process (12). It comprises an individual's motivations, cognitive representations (to visualize what the "future" is), and behavioral components. Seginer and colleagues (33) have stated explicitly the importance of "behavioral components." There are two variables indicating the "behavioral components" – "exploration" and "commitment." The process of exploration helps one to determine the extent to which one's personal abilities, values, environmental circumstances, or social expectations are aligned with the future options (34). The individual is seeking advice and information regarding their future options in this process. "Commitment" results in "a sense of knowing where one is going" (35) and the resolution to pursue a particular option. It is about continuity of the belief and concrete action-taking to pursue the options. Both variables are instrumental to children's and adolescents' future orientation toward future goal achievement.

Future orientation is particularly important in early adolescence (36, 37). During this transitional developmental stage, youths are often confronted with situations where they are required to make choices. For instance, they may be tempted to experiment with sex or drugs, or to choose their peers (38). In face of these situations, the ability to look ahead to the future and speculate how present decisions or behaviors may result in consequences in the future become increasingly vital to successful navigation in this developmental phase. McCabe and Barnett (39) cautioned that, while youths do evaluate the realism of their future plans, particularly in terms of their career development. They, however, lack the skills to generate plausible solutions to overcome obstacles that may interfere with the achievement of their goals, specifically family- or relationship-related goals. Therefore, better communication and more assistance should be provided to help children and adolescents understand what "future" means and guide them to search their pathways.

Future orientation represents the images of the future relating experiences or events subsumed under different life domains (40). Cross-cultural studies have found that adolescents are mainly concerned with career, romantic relationships, and family (e.g., establishing a family with their spouse) domains in life (36). However, most of the studies have primarily focused on adolescents' understanding of future educational or career achievement. This focus is consistent with the findings of "aspirations" and "hopes." Many present intervention programs, as a result, are just exclusively focusing on examining youth's career and educational plans but ignoring the establishment of relationships and family plans. Future research may focus on investigating children and adolescents' perceptions of and the difficulties encountered in relationship-building and establishment of families. Moreover, outcome studies may include variables such as academic achievement and positive psychological and social adjustment.

Resilience

Research on resilience has been heavily focused on developmental psychopathology in the past few decades. Resilience has gained much attention from research about positive psychology in recent decades and there is a shift of focus to investigating the relationships between resilience and positive youth development (41, 42). It relates to the concepts "optimism," "faith and hope," and "sense of self" (43). Resilience is characterized by one's inclination to overcome rather than succumb to the effects of risks (37, 44). It emphasizes individuals' strengths rather than vulnerability (45). Resilience is exhibited when one acknowledges the presence of risks, adversities, and challenges and willingly adapts or copes with the situation (46, 47). Resilience is understood to be a result of negotiations between individuals who identify themselves as physiologically, psychologically and mentally healthy and their environments in conditions collectively viewed as adverse (45). In other words, an individual's resilience develops in response to challenges, not in their absence, and the individual has then the capacity and capability to face these challenges.

In the comprehensive literature review of Khanlou and Wray (45), resilience is regarded as a multidimensional concept and is a) a process (rather than a single event), b) a continuum (rather than a binary outcome), and c) likely a global concept with specific dimensions. When resilience is perceived as a "process," it develops over time; depending on the interactions between systems involved, the time period can vary across individuals and settings. As a continuum, the same individual can be in different parts of the continuum of resilience depending on the available support systems (e.g., family, school or community) and challenges faced over time.

Resilience can also be experienced as a global process, and there are specific domains of resilience such as academic resilience or social resilience. Lee et al. (42), summarized the existing literature on the definition of resilience in the review, and proposed that three components, "capacity," "process" and "results," should be encompassed in defining the concept. The concepts "capacity" and "process" share some commonalities with the propositions of Khanlou and Wray on "process" and "continuum." The component "result" is defined as the positive and beneficial outcomes resulting from successfully navigating stressful events (42).

Although the concept "resilience" has been investigated and explored for several decades, Alperstein and Raman (48) observed that research has predominantly focused on physical health and less on determinants of mental health concerns at the macro level, "and even less on emotional well-being and enhancing 'coping' or promoting resilience" (p. 269). Thus, it is recommended to conduct research on resilience and evaluations on interventions of the role of resilience in promoting mental health.

Beliefs in the future

There is scarce literature conceptualizing "beliefs in the future" in both Western and Chinese contexts. Catalano et al. (41) defined "beliefs in the future" as "an internalization of hope and optimism about possible outcomes" (41), in which the concept "beliefs in the future" entails the concepts of "hope" and "optimism." Based on the definition suggested by Catalano et al. (41), Sun and Lau (49) stated that the concept includes two components, which are a) goal-directed thoughts, that is, to set achievable goals and pursue the goals with possible pathways; and b) goal-directed motivation, which is self-efficacy derived from positive self-appraisal. The thoughts and motivations reciprocally influence each other and would "rejuvenate" (3) when the goals are successfully achieved. In addition, these two components encompass some common features with the concepts of "hope" (the goals for the individual), "aspirations" (the motivation of pursuit) and "future orientation" (the wish that the individual would like to accomplish). The concept "beliefs in the future" has been used interchangeably with the concepts "hope" and "future orientation."

The above discussion outlines a brief conceptual review of the concept of dream and the related constructs. The review shows that most of the concepts share some common features conceptually yet each concept has also some unique underpinnings. The concepts under review are thus evidently all crucial to children's and adolescents' development.

QUESTIONS TO BE CONSIDERED AND FUTURE RESEARCH DIRECTIONS

According to Wu, Leung and Shek (4), with reference to the concept of dream and related constructs, several categories of questions should be raised for consideration. The first category of questions is related to the basic concept of dream and the related constructs. There are several questions that researchers and practitioners should consider:

1) What are the psychological, physiological and social processes, steps, and paths that lead to the achievement of a dream? If so, how and when?
2) What is the importance of practicality in leading children successfully to their dreams?
3) Should the "appropriateness" of a dream be considered? If so, at what stage of development?
4) Is it advisable to do a reality check on dreams of youth? Does this limit their future orientation or keep them from experiencing disappointment?

Regarding the factors that influence the development of dreams and related constructs, several questions should be asked:

1) What motivates students to have a dream?
2) At what age is it likely to see future orientation in children? What contributes to delays or absence of future orientation?
3) Should aptitude and intellectual ability be considered in helping a child achieve his or her dream? If so, at what stage of development?
4) What barriers does a youth normally run into when trying to achieve their dreams? When they face challenges/barriers, what are the components that help these young people overcome them?
5) How can teachers and schools support their students? What are their roles?
6) How can peers support one of their own? What is their role?
7) Do parents influence youth's dreams? How can parents support their children? What is their role? What happens if the child's dream is not in line with the parent's dream for their child? How to come to a resolution?

Concerning the consequences of having dreams and related attributes, the following questions should be asked:

1) Why is it good to have a dream? What are the general and specific benefits?
2) What happens if one does not have a dream?
3) How will the youth's dream help other people, the community and the society at large?

Finally, for the existing interventions from the Western and Chinese contexts, the first two questions are raised:

1) Should there be active intervention to shift the focus of a child's dreams? If so, at what stage of development?

2) Is the assessment of talents, ability, passion and interest important in helping children achieve their dreams? If so, how this should be done?

As we focus on the concept of dream and the related constructs in this paper, we will discuss the first category of questions. For the other categories of questions, they will be addressed in the second paper and third paper. Regarding the first question (i.e., processes and pathways), the review conducted by Wu, Leung and Shek (4) shows that there are very few developmental models to state clearly the processes, steps, or paths that lead to the development of a dream. In fact, there are unique ways for each individual to achieve his or her dreams, which might be influenced by the psychological, physiological and social factors.

For the other questions, most of the existing literature emphasizes the *possibility* of the children and adolescents in searching for their own dreams or aspirations. Some scholars cautioned the "practicality," with a strong emphasis on academic excellence, or "appropriateness" (for example, the parental or societal expectations) might hinder the motivation and willingness of the Chinese youth to search for their own future. Although some of the children or adolescents will evaluate the realism of their future plans, the search for the possibility is the "essence" perceived by the youth when they search for future dreams and the "reality check" might limit their orientation.

In view of the paucity of research on the concept of dream and related constructs, Wu, Leung and Shek (4) proposed several directions for future research in terms of theoretical conceptualization of the concept of dream and the related constructs. First, there is scarce literature conceptualizing the idea "dream," yet the usage of "dream" related to the concepts of "hope," "aspirations," and "future orientation" is immensely common in the media. The interchangeable usage of "dream" and "hope" or "aspirations" suggests that theoretically there is a need to provide a clearer differentiation among the concepts. Empirical studies may be conducted to delineate the unique psychological constructs that differentiate the concepts from each other. The theoretical and research literature on "dream" reflects little consensus about definitions, with scarce well-developed conceptualization and operationalization of the concept. We believe that concerted attention could be given to justify strategies used to operationalize the concept and it is crucial for the investigators to exercise caution in the use of terminologies.

Second, earlier conceptualizations and research on the constructs have focused predominantly on the individual. In more recent years, conceptualizations and investigations have moved beyond the level of the individual to include other influential factors such as peers and parents. Future research may adopt an ecological approach to examine factors on the individual, family, school, and community levels that may impact on children's and adolescents' hope, dreams, aspirations, and future orientation. This research would allow for more holistic and comprehensive theoretical models and shed light on the psychological underpinnings of the constructs.

ACKNOWLEDGMENTS

The current project was financially supported by The Bao Bao Bear Care Foundation Limited. The materials in this chapter are based on a paper published in the *International Journal on Disability and Human Development* 2017;16(4) issue.

REFERENCES

[1] Benson PL. All kids are our kids: What communities must do to raise caring and responsible children and adolescents. San Francisco, CA: Jossey-Bass, 2006.

[2] Catalano RF, Hawkins JD, Berglund ML, Pollard JA, Arthur MW. Prevention science and positive youth development: Competitive or cooperative frameworks? J Adolesc Health 2002;31(6):230-9.

[3] Sun RCF, Shek DTL. Beliefs in the future as a positive youth development construct: A conceptual review. ScientificWorldJournal 2012;12. DOI: 10.1100/2012/527038.

[4] Wu FKY, Leung H, Shek DTL. Collaborative research report on "Literature review on hope and aspirations in children and adolescents." [Unpublished manuscript] Hong

Kong: Department of Applied Social Sciences, The Hong Kong Polytechnic University, 2015.

[5] Juvakka T, Kylmä J. Hope in adolescents with cancer. Eur J Oncol Nurs 2009;13(3):193-9.

[6] Valle MF, Huebner ES, Suldo SM. An analysis of hope as a psychological strength. J Sch Psychol 2006;44(5):393-406.

[7] Freud S. Introductory lectures on psycho-analysis. S.E., 15/16. London: Hogarth Press, 1916-1917.

[8] Yohani S. Nurturing hope in refugee children during early years of post-war adjustment. Child Youth Serv Rev 2010;32(6):865-73.

[9] Li J. "Please let children develop through pursing their dreams": A study of children's moral development in Hongze county primary school. Jiangsu Educ Res 2013;17:30-3.

[10] Quaglia RJ, Cobb CD. Toward a theory of student aspirations. J Res Rural Educ 1996;12(3):127-32.

[11] Rojewski JW. Occupational aspirations: Constructs, meanings, and application. In: Brown SD, Lent RW, eds. Career development and counseling: Putting theory and research to work. New York: John Wiley, 2005:131-54.

[12] Nurmi JE. How do adolescents see their future? A review of the development of future orientation and planning. Dev Rev 1991;11(1):1-59.

[13] Gil-Flores J, Padilla-Carmona MT, Suárez-Ortega M. Influence of gender, educational attainment and family environment on the educational aspirations of secondary school students. Educ Rev 2011;63(3):345-63.

[14] Hill NE, Castellino DR, Lansford JE, Nowlin P, Dodge KA, Bates JE, Pettit GS. Parent academic involvement as related to school behavior, achievement, and aspirations: Demographic variations across adolescence. Child Dev 2004;75(5):1491-509.

[15] Marjoribanks K. Family contexts, individual characteristics, proximal settings, and adolescents' aspirations. Psychol Rep 2002;91:769-79.

[16] Patton W, Creed P. Occupational aspirations and expectations of Australian adolescents. Aust J Career Dev 2007;16(1):46-59.

[17] Sirin SR, Diewer MA, Jackson LR, Gonsalves L, Howell A. Future aspirations of urban adolescents: A person-in-context model. Int J Qual Stud Educ 2004;17:437-56.

[18] Salmela-Aro K, Kiuru N, Leskinen E, Nurmi JE. School burnout inventory (SBI) reliability and validity. Eur J Psychol Assess 2009;25(1):48-57.

[19] Snyder CR, Harris C, Anderson JR, Holleran SA, Irving LM, Sigmon ST, et al. The will and the ways: development and validation of an individual-differences measure of hope. J Pers Soc Psychol 1991;60(4):570-85.

[20] Snyder CR. Hypothesis: There is hope. In: Snyder CR, ed. Handbook of hope: Theory, measures, and applications. San Diego, CA: Academic Press, 2000:3-21.

[21] Lloyd TJ, Hastings R. Hope as a psychological resilience factor in mothers and fathers of children with intellectual disabilities. J Intellect Disabil Res 2009;53(12):957-68.

[22] Scheier MF, Carver CS. Optimism, coping, and health: Assessment and implications of generalized outcome expectancies. Health Psychol 1985;4(3):219-47.

[23] Bandura A. Self-efficacy mechanism in human agency. Am Psychol 1982;37(2):122-47.

[24] Bailey TC, Eng W, Frisch MB, Snyder CR. Hope and optimism as related to life satisfaction. J Posit Psychol 2007;2:168-75.

[25] Edwards LM, Ong AD, Lopez SJ. Hope measurement in Mexican American youth. Hisp J Behav Sci 2007;29(2):225-41.

[26] Truitt M, Biesecker B, Capone G, Bailey T, Erby L. The role of hope in adaptation to uncertainty: The experience of caregivers of children with down syndrome. Patient Educ Couns 2012;87(2):233-8.

[27] Onwuegbuzie AJ, Snyder CR. Relations between hope and graduate students' coping strategies for studying and examination-taking. Psychol Rep 2000;86(3):803-6.

[28] Peterson SJ, Gerhardt MW, Rode JC. Hope, learning goals, and task performance. Pers Individ Diff 2006;40(6):1099-109.

[29] Callina KS, Johnson SK, Buckingham MH, Lerner RM. Hope in context: Developmental profiles of trust, hopeful future expectations, and civic engagement across adolescence. J Youth Adolesc 2014;43(6):869-83.

[30] Te Riele K. Philosophy of hope: concepts and applications for working with marginalized youth. J Youth Stud 2010;13(1):35-46.

[31] Padilla-Walker LM, Hardy SA, Christensen KJ. Adolescent hope as a mediator between parent-child connectedness and adolescent outcomes. J Early Adolesc 2011;31(6):853-79.

[32] Valle MF, Huebner ES, Suldo SM. An analysis of hope as a psychological strength. J Sch Psychol 2006;44(5), 393-406.

[33] Seginer R, Shoyer S. How mothers affect adolescents' future orientation: A two-source analysis. Jpn Psychol Res 2012;54(3):310-20.

[34] Lewin K. Field theory and experiment in social psychology: Concepts and methods. Am J Sociol 1939;44(6):868-96.

[35] Erikson EH. Identity: Youth and crisis. New York: WW Norton, 1968.

[36] Greene AL. Future-time perspective in adolescence: The present of things future revisited. J Youth Adolesc 1986;15(2):99-113.

[37] Rutter M. Psychosocial resilience and protective mechanisms. Am J Orthopsychiatry 1987;57(3):316-31.

[38] Dryfoos JG. Adolescents at risk: Prevalence and prevention. New York: Oxford University Press, 1990.

[39] McCabe KM, Barnett, D. The relation between familial factors and the future orientation of urban, African American sixth graders. J Child Fam Stud 2000;9(4):491-508.

[40] Nuttin J, Lens W. Future time perspective and motivation: Theory and research method. Leuven: University Press and Lawrence Erlbaum Associates, 1985.

[41] Catalano RF, Berglund ML, Ryan JA, Lonczak HS, Hawkins JD. Positive youth development in the United States: Research findings on evaluations of positive youth development programs. Ann Am Acad Pol Soc Sci 2004;591(1):98-124.

[42] Lee TY, Cheung CK, Kwong WM. Resilience as a positive youth development construct: a conceptual review. ScientificWorldJournal 2012;12. DOI: 10.1100/2012/390450.

[43] Edward K-l. Resilience: A protector from depression. J Am Psychiatr Nurses Assoc 2005;11(4):241-3.

[44] Ager A. Annual Research Review: Resilience and child well-being-public policy implications. J Child Psychol Psychiatry 2013;54(4):488-500.

[45] Khanlou N, Wray R. A whole community approach toward child and youth resilience promotion: A review of resilience literature. Int J Ment Health Addict 2014;12(1):64-79.

[46] Masten AS. Resilience in developing systems: Progress and promise as the fourth wave rises. Dev Psychopathol 2007;19(03):921-30.

[47] Masten A, Herbers J, Cutuli J, Lafavor T. Promoting competence and resilience in the school context. Prof School Couns 2008;12(2):76-84.

[48] Alperstein G, Raman S. Promoting mental health and emotional well-being among children and youth: A role for community child health? Child: Care, Health Dev 2003;29(4):269-74.

[49] Sun RCF, Lau PSY. Beliefs in the future as a positive youth development construct: Conceptual bases and implications for curriculum development. Int J Adolesc Med Health 2006;18(3):409-16.

In: Soft Skills and Aspirations … ISBN: 978-1-53614-092-7
Editors: Daniel TL Shek, et al.

Chapter 7

HOPE, ASPIRATIONS AND RESILIENCE IN CHILDREN AND ADOLESCENTS

Hildie Leung*[1]*, PhD, Florence KY Wu*[1]*, EdD and Daniel TL Shek*[1-5,*]*, PhD, FHKPS, BBS, JP

[1]Department of Applied Social Sciences, The Hong Kong Polytechnic University, Hong Kong, PR China
[2]Centre for Innovative Programmes for Adolescents and Families, The Hong Kong Polytechnic University, Hong Kong, PR China
[3]Kiang Wu Nursing College of Macau, Macau, PR China
[4]Department of Social Work, East China Normal University, PR China
[5]Division of Adolescent Medicine, Department of Pediatrics, Kentucky Children's Hospital, University of Kentucky College of Medicine, Lexington, Kentucky, US

ABSTRACT

Hope, aspirations, and resilience are important developmental assets for children and adolescents. Based on the existing Western and Chinese literature, this chapter aims to identify instruments used to assess hope, aspirations, resilience, and conceptually related constructs as well as

[*] Corresponding Author Email: daniel.shek@polyu.edu.hk.

antecedents of the constructs in adolescents. A systematic literature search in the major databases was conducted, resulting in 223 articles, with 144 being retrieved from international databases and 79 from the China's database were included in this review. Findings revealed that the majority of existing scales were developed predominantly in the West and there were few validated Chinese hope and aspirations scales. Indigenous measures were also not identified in the literature. In terms of antecedents of dreams and related constructs, predictors at different levels including the personal, family, school, and community were found. Implications on the development of hope-based interventions and recommendations for future research are discussed.

INTRODUCTION

Psychologists have long been preoccupied with human pathology prior to the dawn of the positive psychology movement. In 1998, Seligman argued that instead of merely focusing on studying what went wrong with individuals, a paradigmatic shift should be made to investigate what is non-pathological. Based on this premise, he established the field of positive psychology as the scientific study of factors that enable individuals to thrive, lead fulfilling lives, and achieve optimal human functioning (1). In the area of developmental psychology, scholars shared the same sentiments and articulated the benefits of adopting a positive youth development approach to study and promote developmental assets among youngsters (2).

Among the developmental constructs, beliefs in the future (future aspirations, future orientations), hope, and resilience have been identified as important personal strengths for positive youth development (3, 4). Beliefs in the future is defined as an internalization of hope and optimism about possible outcomes (5). More specifically, hope is defined as "the process of thinking about one's goals, along with the motivation to move toward (agency) and the ways to achieve (pathways) those goals" (6). According to Sun and Shek (4), "promotion of beliefs in the future for positive youth development deserves greater attention… noting that hope and optimism are two core components of beliefs in the future, it is necessary to help adolescents to internalize both hope and optimism" (4). However, before this can be done, there is a need to examine 1) the theoretical concepts of the hope, aspirations, and resilience; 2) how the concepts are measured among youths; 3) its antecedents; and 4) the outcomes. The conceptual review of the concepts along with findings from outcomes studies have been reported elsewhere. The present review attempted to identify instruments used to assess children and adolescent hope, aspirations, resilience, and conceptually related constructs as well as the antecedents of the constructs in the existing literature. It is hoped that this systematic review would allow for critical appraisal of existing studies and guide future research and hope-based interventions.

Review of the Literature

Studies published in journals spanning from 1980 to 2015 were included in the review. Articles were identified via online databases, including PsycINFO, Academic Search Premier, Web of Science, EBSCOhost database, and China's database CAJ Full-text Database. The search terms "dreams", "hope", "aspirations", "future orientation", "resilience", "beliefs in the future", "children", and "adolescents" were used. Articles which met the following inclusion criteria were included in the review: 1) the focus of the study is the youth population, i.e., individuals aged between 6 and 18; 2) the study addressed the conceptualization of hope, aspirations, resilience or its related concepts; 3) the study examines the development or validation of measurement tools of hope, aspirations, resilience, or its related concepts; and 4) the study was conducted in the Western context or in China. A total of 223 articles, with 144 being retrieved from international databases and 79 from the China's database met the criteria and were included in the present review.

Measuring hope, aspirations, resilience and related concepts

Several measurements on hope were identified in the literature review. In the West, commonly used instruments include the Adult Dispositional Hope

Scale (7), Children's Hope Scale (8), Beck Hopelessness Scale (9), Hopelessness Scale for Children (10), and Herth Hope Index (11). In China, the Chinese versions of the Adult Dispositional Hope Scale and Children's Hope Scale are the most widely administered instruments. Several observations were generated regarding the identified instruments. First, in terms of the target population, scales such as Herth Hope Index were initially developed for physically ill patients. As such, its generalizability to the general adolescent population may be limited. Second, some of the measures lack assessment of goal-setting and goal-pursuit which are particularly relevant to hope-based interventions that aim to enhance students' motivations to pursue their dreams (12). Thus, there may be a need to include and adapt items from scales such as the Miller Hope Scale (13) and the Adult Dispositional Hope Scale (7) which assess goal identification and achievement. Third, strengths of the commonly used scales such as the Adult Dispositional Hope Scale and the Children's Hope Scale are that they have been validated in the Chinese context.

Assessment of aspirations

In terms of assessing aspirations among children and adolescents, studies have revealed that the concept is measured in terms of two main dimensions, i.e., educational aspirations and career aspirations. For educational aspirations, most scholars (14-16) used a single-item to assess students' educational aspirations by inviting them to indicate by a certain age (e.g., 30 years old), "*What level of education do you hope to hold?*" with options such as 0 (*no further education planned*), 9 (*PhD or equivalent*), to 10 (*MD, LLB, JD, DDS, or equivalent*). Some scholars also used other related items or scales to shed light on adolescents' academic aspirations such as their attitudes in school (17) or the amount of time they spend on their assignments or studies (18). Given that there are few validated scales to measure educational aspirations in both Western and Chinese literature, there is a need to develop and validate scales to measure youths' educational aspirations which include related concepts such as educational motivation, beliefs, self-efficacy, and associated behaviors.

Similar to the measurement of future orientation, there are few validated studies on career aspirations measurement. A commonly used instrument is the Career Aspirations Scale (CAS) (19), which includes three subscales (Leadership and Achievement, Job Satisfaction, and Continue Education). Other scholars assessed occupational aspirations of students by asking young people to indicate their preferred occupations using a single item such as "*Nearly everyone of your age has some sort of idea of what they will want to do in life. Here is a list of the types of jobs/careers/professions for which various amounts of training are necessary. How about your choice(s)?*" Researchers then categorized the data based on their research question (e.g., professional or managerial occupations vs. skilled, semi-skilled, or unskilled jobs) (e.g., 20).

In addition to the widespread categorization of career and educational aspirations, Kasser and Ryan (21) developed the Aspirations Index to assess both intrinsic (e.g., personal growth, relatedness, community service, and intellectual-aesthetic growth) and extrinsic (e.g., financial success, attractiveness, fame, power, and health) aspirations or life-goals. For studies conducted in mainland China, students' vocational aspirations were assessed using The Occupations List – Chinese Version (OLC) (22) based on Holland's Vocational Preference Inventory (23, 24). While instruments measuring students' interests provide useful information, it is argued that "expressed interest in a profession has been shown to be equal to or to exceed interest inventories in predicting a person's future occupation" (20, p. 212). Therefore, future studies may include both interest and expressed interest items to better understand youth's career aspirations. In addition, it may also be useful to measure students' difficulties in career decision-making with scales such as the Career Decision-making Difficulties Questionnaire (25) which will shed light on what to include in interventions to cater for the youths' needs.

Assessment of future orientation

Compared with other concepts in the present literature review (e.g., hope and resilience) there were relatively fewer scales measuring future orientation. Many scholars merely used a few items to measure future orientation such as "*I have plans for my future*", or "*I am doing things now that will help me in the future*" (26). The Future Orientation Questionnaire adopted by Nurmi et al. (27) and Seginer et al. (28) focuses on three future orientation domains (i.e., higher education, career, and marriage). Seginer and colleagues' scale provides a comprehensive assessment as it taps behavioral, cognitive, and motivational components of future orientation. Furthermore, the Life Orientation Test (29) was also used for children and adolescents. Sun and Shek (4) reported that the psychometrically validated Hope Scale (7) and the Life Orientation Test have been found to have convergent validity which lends support to the interrelatedness of the concepts of hope, optimism, and future orientation.

Another commonly used measurement of future orientation is the Future Orientation Questionnaire (30) with open-ended questions where students were invited to list their hoped-for and feared selves. The interviewers then invited respondents to state the age they thought they could achieve their hoped-for selves, and also the extent they believed they could achieve their hoped-for selves (see 31). In fact, many of the studies used a qualitative approach (e.g., interviews) to assess children's and adolescents' future orientation.

Assessment of resilience

Several observations can be drawn from the review. First, many resilience scales were initially developed for clinical practice as a measure of stress coping ability among adults or adolescents who have experienced traumatic events, rather than measuring the profiles of children and adolescents in general. Second, in terms of methodological concerns, some scales yielded relatively low Cronbach alpha values (e.g., Ego Resilience scale) (32) which raise questions about the internal consistency of the items. Third, there is an absence of a psychometrically robust measure of resilience for young children. Fourth, few scales included items to assess the availability of assets and resources that facilitate resilience. Therefore, in order to gain a comprehensive picture of children's and adolescents' resilience, particularly if it were to shed light on intervention needs, the instrument should be able to assess a range of protective mechanisms across domains that contribute to resilience (33). For instance, Donnon and Hammond's (34) Youth Resiliency: Assessing Developmental Strengths examines intrinsic and extrinsic protective factors among the youth.

PREDICTORS OF HOPE, ASPIRATIONS, AND RESILIENCE AMONG YOUTHS

Developmental systems theory advocates the inherent plasticity of human development. That is, individuals have the potential for systematic change throughout their lifespan. These changes result from mutual interactions between the developing individual and his/her biological, psychological, as well as the ecological context (e.g., family, peers, school, community, and culture) (35). Indeed, a review of literature on the development of aspirations and hope among children and adolescents revealed factors at different levels (i.e., individual, familial, school, and community) have an impact on the development of the different constructs.

Individual factors

On a personal level, gender and identity have been found to be predictors. Regarding the impact of gender on aspirations, existing findings in the West remain mixed. While some studies showed that female high school students were more future-oriented than their male counterparts on both career and education (36), other studies showed few gender differences in future orientation (37). What is more interesting is that female and male adolescents had different career aspirations. Ashby and Schoon (38) found that a significantly higher proportion of teenage girls aspired to professional or managerial positions as compared with teenage boys. In terms of occupational dreams and aspirations, adolescent boys reported higher levels of entrepreneurial orientations (39). Adolescent boys also preferred jobs in which they could be challenged. They aspired to have jobs in fields that are male-dominated (e.g., business management, architecture), whereas girls aspired to careers that are traditionally female-dominated (e.g., elementary school teaching, journalism) (40).

Gender differences were also observed in studies conducted in mainland China. In terms of resilience, studies conducted with Chinese migrant children (41) and university students (42) generally found that females reported higher levels of resilience. However, in a study of adolescents in Chengdu subsequent to the Sichuan earthquake, Yu and colleagues (43) found that male respondents reported higher resilience scores than did females. In Meng and colleagues' (44) study with primary and secondary school students who were affected by AIDS, boys reported higher levels of hope than did girls. In terms of future orientation, generally speaking, female students reported higher levels of future orientation than did male students (45). More specifically, female students held higher levels of aspirations in the educational area, whereas males had higher aspirations in the marriage and family domain (46, 47).

In terms of career aspirations, using Holland's Vocational Preference Inventory (24), Hou and Leung (23) investigated vocational aspirations of Chinese high school students and identified gender differences, which suggested that male students aspired to occupational fields that were Investigative, Enterprising and Artistic (IEA) whereas female students aspired to Artistic, Enterprising and Investigative (AEI) occupations. Moreover, male students considered occupations of higher prestige and of more masculine compared with female students. Similarly, Creed et al. (48) found that Chinese male high school students aspired to Investigative and Enterprising types of occupations, but expected Realistic and Enterprising ones, whereas female students aspired to Enterprising and Conventional types, but expected Conventional and Social ones.

The above findings have important implications for interventions. First, to reconcile the discrepancy between aspirations and expectations, practitioners should focus on helping students to better understand the possible career barriers and enhance their career confidence to overcome those barriers. Second, students should be encouraged to expand their career interests. For instance, students should be encouraged to attend career exploration activities to increase their awareness of diverse career opportunities and different educational or career pathways to achieve their dreams. "The traditional Chinese idea that 'all trades and professions have their masters' could be useful as a 'culture-based' rationale to encourage openness to occupational alternatives" (23). Third, students should be encouraged to give more consideration to careers out of their gender stereotypes.

Besides gender, age has been identified as a factor affecting resilience. It is generally believed that adolescent resilience is a developmental process in which resilience increases with age. Children learn to make use of assets and resources when they are exposed to adversity. Their levels of resilience are enhanced when they successfully overcome low levels of risk, and become prepared to tackle greater challenges (49). However, literature search revealed that there are few studies conducted to specifically examine age differences in the development of hope and aspirations. Steinberg et al. (50) found that younger adolescents had lower levels of future orientation than individuals aged 16 or over. Yet future orientation is a critical issue when children approach adolescence because they are required to reflect, and make detailed plans and realistic evaluations of their ability to reach future goals (51). Scholars have therefore advised that interventions may begin in early high school years to encourage young adolescents to explore their future aspirations (23).

Besides gender and age, self-efficacy is also a personal predictor of future orientation. Self-efficacy in the context of future orientation refers to adolescents' internal beliefs about his/her level of competence and ability to perform well in the future (52). According to studies conducted in the West and China, findings showed a consistent positive relationship between children's and adolescents' self-efficacy and their future orientation. Adolescents with higher levels of self-efficacy reported higher levels of educational aspirations (53, 54). In a study of adolescent vocational students in China, Zong and Li (55) found that students' career decision-making self-efficacy was positively correlated with characteristics of hope such as their way of thinking, will power, and general self-esteem. Indeed, the more efficacious students feel, the more likely they are able to persist in their studies and strive to attain their goals. Bandura et al. (56) also found that children's perceived efficacy influenced their career pursuits. Generally speaking, research findings supported that children's and adolescents' self-efficacy beliefs determine the career aspirations or options that they will consider. As such, interventions may aim to enhance children's and adolescents' self-efficacy. This can be done by 1) providing environments and opportunities that reinforce the probability that the children would experience success due to their own abilities and efforts; 2) empowerment through reinforcing their personal control to increase a sense of ownership and responsibility for their lives; 3) helping children and adolescents to identify their strengths and areas of competence which may be sources for pride and accomplishments; and 4) providing students with chances to showcase their talents and have them valued by significant figures (e.g., peers, parents, and teachers) (57).

Family factors

In terms of socioeconomic status (SES), studies generally showed that well-off adolescents reported higher levels of aspirations compared with their counterparts from low-SES backgrounds (16). Adolescents from higher income families also aspired to more professional jobs and expected to stay in school than those from lower income families. Particularly, teenage girls from higher income families were more likely to value having a job that enabled them to have higher levels of ambition and "aim high" (38). An interesting finding in a recent Australian study showed that adolescents from high SES backgrounds cited interest and passion as motivation for their career choices, whereas their counterparts from low SES cited money as a consideration (58). However, it is noteworthy that the pattern of SES on aspirations is different in studies conducted in China. Jiang (59) found that poorer college students reported higher levels of aspirations than did non-poor students. The author reasoned that this may be due to the increasing Government support allocated to alleviate their financial difficulties, which helped to enhance their self-esteem and motivation to achieve their goals.

Research has also shown that better family functioning was related to higher levels of aspirations and hope among children and adolescents. For instance, supportive and safe parental relationships such as being able to seek help from and to freely communicate with parents helped the youth to maintain their future aspirations (3). Adolescents with supportive parents were more optimistic and hopeful as well (60). Children who perceived their parents as loving and supportive were more willing to develop a trusting and positive attitude towards their future, had more confidence in future success as a result of their contributions, and were more likely to invest to achieve their future goals (61). On the other hand, Chinese American adolescents from families with more intergenerational conflicts reported higher levels of career indecision (62). In China, a study conducted on migrant children also found that parent-child attachment was positively related to children's resilience (41). Zhang and Zhang (46) also found that parent-child communication significantly predicted youths' career achievement planning.

Parenting is also an important determinant of hope and related constructs in adolescents. Scholars found that adolescents' perceived autonomous-accepting parenting was positively associated with their future orientation (37, 63). Adolescents who perceived their parents as warm and accepting reported higher levels of future orientation (52, 61). In Nurmi and Pulliainen's (63) qualitative study, the authors found that for 11-year-olds, those who reported higher parental control were less optimistic about their future. However, for 15-year-olds, the higher level of family discussion they reported, the more optimistic they were about their future. Indeed, it is believed that older adolescents may be more able to articulate their ideas and express their emotions related to future orientation, such as fear or hope (64). Few studies have been conducted to examine the direct relationship between parenting and adolescents' future orientation in China. However, in a cross-cultural study comparing young adolescents from the USA, Canada, and China, Lekes and colleagues (65) found that universally, autonomy-supportive parents were more likely to endorse adolescents' intrinsic life goals (e.g., community-related goals such as improving the world, affiliation, and self-acceptance), which were in turn associated with adolescent well-being and were likely to impact on their future orientation. Wu and Chen (66) also found that parenting impacted on adolescents' resilience. Particularly, maternal emotional warmth significantly predicted college students' resilience, and paternal overprotection had negative effects on resilience.

Parental expectations have also been shown to have a positive relationship with educational aspirations (67). Ashby and Schoon (38) found that teenage career aspirations, ambition value, and educational performance at age 16 all increased with parental educational aspirations of their offspring. It is speculated that parents who have high expectations and aspirations on their children may be more involved in their studies and prioritized educational endeavors. Moreover, they may be more open and willing to discuss and communicate about their child's future. In China, Hou and Leung (23) found that parents expected male students to pursue Investigative (e.g., science-related) occupations, and Enterprising (e.g., business-related) occupations were also preferred for both sons and daughters. Chinese parents often expect their children to work in scientific and professional fields and place a high value on prestige in job selection, especially for their sons (68). These expectations are likely to impact on students' future career aspirations.

In addition, as Confucian values on family obligations are strong in the Mainland, individuals are expected to provide support, assistance, and respect to family members. Fuligni and Zhang (69) found that Chinese adolescents reported a strong sense of family obligation, and this was associated with higher levels of academic motivation. However, counter intuitively, family obligation was not associated with students' educational aspirations.

Given the importance of parental expectations and aspirations on the development of children's and adolescents' aspirations, some recommendations are suggested: 1) interventions may be designed to educate parents on "reasonable" and "realistic" parental expectations; 2) counselors and teachers may include parental participation in career exploration events; and 3) assistance should be given to students who experience internal conflicts, anxieties or tensions between self-actualization and fulfilling family obligations. Students may be equipped with negotiation, conflict resolution, cooperation, assertiveness, and communication skills so that parents may recognize students' aspirations without feeling that they are disrespected or disobeyed (70).

School factors

Research showed that high achieving adolescents reported higher future aspirations (16). A plausible reason is that high achieving students have better self-concept and higher levels of self-efficacy, which have been found to have positive impacts on their future orientation. Some scholars argued that comparative effect of academic achievement may be present in school, where students compare their own academic performance to that of their peers. Students who have lower academic achievement may have a pessimistic future orientation and establish lower aspirations due to a sense of hopelessness and incompetence (71). Furthermore, the authors found that a school climate of future orientation amplified the protective effects of adolescents' future orientation on problem behaviors.

Besides, adolescents who reported being more connected to their schools reported higher levels of future orientation. These students often have better academic performance and high-quality relationships with their teachers and peers. It is reasoned that when adolescents feel more competent at school, they are more ready, willing, and confident to think and plan for their future (72). Interventions may target at enhancing students' sense of belonging in the school context and encourage supportive peer relationships and student-teacher relationships.

Community factors

Strayhorn (16) found support for neighborhood effects on Black adolescents' educational aspirations where suburban adolescents reported higher levels of educational aspiration than did rural samples. In fact, adolescents' achievement and aspirations have been shown to be correlated with educational histories and aspirations of their peers (73). It is argued that values and beliefs may be reinforced among peers in a neighborhood or system. Therefore, to maximize the positive neighborhood effect, it is recommended that resources may be devoted to establishing learning communities. For instance, after-school programs may be developed to help students better prepare for university or tutoring classes may be arranged for low-achieving students especially in less resourceful communities.

CONCLUSION

Based on a comprehensive literature review on the existing measurements and antecedent studies of hope, aspirations, resilience and related concepts on children and adolescents, the following observations and recommendations were put forth. In terms of scale development, there are few validated scales measuring future orientation and aspirations, especially in mainland China. Among the validated scales, such as resilience and hope measures, majority of them were developed by scholars in the West. Therefore, if studies were to be conducted on children and adolescents in mainland China, indigenous measures that are cultural-specific should be developed or adapted with reference to the Chinese cultural characteristics (e.g., emphasis on family and relationships). Regarding findings from studies on the antecedents, factors on the personal, family, school, and community levels that may impact on children's and adolescents' development of resilience, hope, and aspirations in both the Western and Chinese contexts have been identified. It is recommended that efforts to promote the development of hope and aspirations should take into consideration the risk and protective factors at each level and adopt a holistic approach to address them.

While the review provides an integrative coverage on existing literature in the area of youth hope and aspirations from both the Western and Chinese contexts, a limitation is that only published journal articles were included in the review. Unpublished research such as dissertations, book chapters, and conference papers were excluded. However, given that the aim of the present review is to provide a comprehensive picture of where current research stands, particularly those positioned to influence knowledge development as well as instruments used in the existing literature. Thus, we believe that only rigorous studies that have been published in peer-reviewed journals should be included. As the field develops, a more complete review may include unpublished studies as well as findings from other Asian contexts.

ACKNOWLEDGMENTS

The current project was financially supported by The Bao Bao Bear Care Foundation Limited. The materials in this paper are based on a paper published in the *International Journal on Disability and Human Development* 2017;16(4) issue.

REFERENCES

[1] Seligman ME, Csikszentmihalyi M. Special issue on happiness, excellence, and optimal human functioning. Am Psychol 2000;55(1):5-183.

[2] Catalano RF, Hawkins JD, Berglund ML, Pollard JA, Arthur MW. Prevention science and positive youth development: Competitive or cooperative frameworks? J Adolesc Health 2002;31(6):230-9.

[3] McCoy H, Bowen EA. Hope in the social environment: Factors affecting future aspirations and school self-efficacy for youth in urban environments. Child Adolesc Soc Work J 2015;32(2):131-41.
[4] Sun RCF, Shek DTL. Beliefs in the future as a positive youth development construct: A conceptual review. ScientificWorldJournal; 2012. Article ID 527038, 8 pages. doi: 10.1100/2012/527038.
[5] Catalano RF, Berglund ML, Ryans JA, Lonczak HS, Hawkins JD. Positive youth development in the United States: Research findings on evaluations of positive youth development programs. Washington, DC: Office of Assistant Secretary for Planning and Evaluation, 1998. URL: http://dx.doi.org/10.1100/2012/527038
[6] Snyder CR. Conceptualizing, measuring, and nurturing hope. J Couns Dev 1995;73(3):355-60.
[7] Snyder CR, Harris C, Anderson JR, Holleran SA, Irving LM, Sigmon ST, et al. The will and the ways: Development and validation of an individual-differences measure of hope. J Pers Soc Psychol 1991;60(4):570-85.
[8] Snyder CR, Hoza B, Pelham WE, Rapoff M, Ware L, Danovsky M, et al. The development and validation of the Children's Hope Scale. J Pediatr Psychol 1997; 22(3):399-421.
[9] Beck AT, Steer RA. Beck Hopelessness Scale manual. San Antonio, TX: Psychological corporation, 1988.
[10] Kazdin AE, Rodgers A, Colbus D. The Hopelessness Scale for children: Psychometric characteristics and concurrent validity. J Consult Clin Psych 1986;54(2):241-5.
[11] Herth K. Development and refinement of an instrument to measure hope. Sch Inq Nurs Pract 1991;5(1):39-51. https://search.proquest.com/docview/893000239?pq-origsite=gscholar
[12] Schrank B, Bird V, Rudnick A, Slade M. Determinants, self-management strategies and interventions for hope in people with mental disorders: Systematic search and narrative review. Soc Sci Med 2012;74(4):554-64.
[13] Miller JF, Powers MJ. Development of an instrument to measure hope. Nurs Res 1988;37(1):6-10.
[14] Carranza FD, You S, Chhuon V, Hudley C. Mexican American adolescents' academic achievement and aspirations: The role of perceived parental educational involvement, acculturation, and self-esteem. Adolescence 2009;44(174):313-33.
[15] Carter DF. A dream deferred? Examining the degree aspirations of African American and White college students. New York: Taylor Francis, 2001.
[16] Strayhorn TL. Different folks, different hopes: The educational aspirations of black males in urban, suburban, and rural high schools. Urban Educ 2009;44(6):710-31. http://dx.doi.org/10.1177/0042085908322705.
[17] McCoach DB, Siegle D. The school attitude assessment survey-revised: A new instrument to identify academically able students who underachieve. Educ Psychol Meas 2003;63(3):414-29.

[18] Huang SYL. Learning environments at higher education institutions: Relationships with academic aspirations and satisfaction. Learn Environ Res 2012;15(3):363-78.

[19] O'Brien KM. Career aspiration scale. College Park, MD: Department of Psychology, University of Maryland, 1992.

[20] Schoon I, Polek E. Teenage career aspirations and adult career attainment: The role of gender, social background and general cognitive ability. Int J Behav Dev 2011;35(3):210-7.

[21] Kasser T, Ryan RM. Further examining the American dream: Differential correlates of intrinsic and extrinsic goals. Pers Soc Psychol B 1996;22(3):280-7.

[22] Leung SA, Harmon LW. Individual and sex differences in the zone of acceptable alternatives. J Couns Psychol 1990;37(2):153.

[23] Hou ZJ, Leung SA. Vocational aspirations of Chinese high school students and their parents' expectations. J Vocat Behav 2011;79(2):349-60.

[24] Holland JL. Manual for the vocational preference inventory. Odessa, FL: Psychological Assessment Resources, 1985.

[25] Gati I, Saka N. High school students' career-related decision-making difficulties. J Couns Dev 2001;79(3):331-40.

[26] Peters RJ, Tortolero SR, Johnson RJ, Addy RC, Markham CM, Escobar-Chaves SL, et al. The relationship between future orientation and street substance use among Texas alternative school students. Am J Addict 2005;14(5):478-85.

[27] Nurmi JE, Seginer R, Poole M. Future-orientation questionnaire. Helsinki, Finland: Department of Psychology, University of Helsinki, 1990.

[28] Seginer R, Shoyer S, Hossessi R, Tannous H. Adolescent family and peer relationships: Does culture matter? New Dir Child Adolesc Dev 2007;116:83-99.

[29] Scheier MF, Carver CS. Optimism, coping, and health: Assessment and implications of generalized outcome expectancies. Health Psychol 1985;4(3):219-47.

[30] Trommsdorff G, Lamm H, Schmidt RW. A longitudinal study of adolescents' future orientation (time perspective). J Youth Adolesc 1979;8(2):131-47.

[31] Yowell CM. Possible selves and future orientation: Exploring hopes and fears of Latino boys and girls. J Early Adolesc 2000;20(3):245-80.

[32] Bromley E, Johnson JG, Cohen P. Personality strengths in adolescence and decreased risk of developing mental health problems in early adulthood. Compr Psychiatry 2006;47(4): 315-24.

[33] Windle G, Bennett KM, Noyes J. A methodological review of resilience measurement scales. Health Qual Life Outcomes 2011;9(8):1-18.

[34] Donnon T, Hammond W. Understanding the relationship between resiliency and bullying in adolescence: An assessment of youth resiliency from five urban junior high schools. Child Adolesc Psychiatr Clin N Am 2007;16(2):449-71.

[35] Lerner RM, Lerner JV, Almerigi JB, Theokas C, Phelps E, Gestsdottir S, et al. Positive youth development, participation in community youth development programs, and community contributions of fifth-grade adolescents findings from the

first wave of the 4-H study of positive youth development. J Early Adolesc 2005;25(1):17-71.

[36] Kolesovs A. Domain-specific and general future orientation of high school students in Latvia under socioeconomic changes. Int J Psychol: Biopsychosoc App 2013;12:71-83. URL: https://eltalpykla.vdu.lt/1/31868.

[37] Seginer R, Vermulst A, Shoyer S. The indirect link between perceived parenting and adolescent future orientation: A multiple-step model. Int J Behav Dev 2004;28(4):365-78.

[38] Ashby JS, Schoon I. Career success: The role of teenage career aspirations, ambition value and gender in predicting adult social status and earnings. J Vocat Behav 2010;77(3):350-60.

[39] Schmitt-Rodermund E, Vondracek FW. Occupational dreams, choices and aspirations: Adolescents' enterpreneurial prospects and orientations. J Adolesc 2002;25(1):65-78. doi: http://dx.doi.org/10.1006/jado.2001.0449.

[40] Nikolayenko O. Adolescents' hopes for personal, local, and global future: Insights from Ukraine. Youth Soc 2011;43(1):64-89. doi: http://dx.doi.org/10.1177/0044118X09351281.

[41] Mao XJ, Wang ZH. Migrant children's attachment to their parents and its effect on their resilience. Chinese J Spec Educ 2013;153(3):50-5.

[42] Han L, Liao CJ, Zheng Y. Status of spiritual belief and psychological resilience and their correlation among university students. Chinese J Pub Health 2014;30(003):275-8.

[43] Yu XN, Lau JT, Mak WW, Zhang J, Lui WW. Factor structure and psychometric properties of the Connor-Davidson Resilience Scale among Chinese adolescents. Compre Psychiatry 2011;52(2):218-24.

[44] Meng QF, Zhong YH, Tian YH. Relationship of subjective well-being and belief in a just world and hope of AIDS-affected children. Chinese Ment Health J 2015;29(1):28-33.

[45] Wang Q. The relationship between future orientation and self-esteem among college students. J Neijiang Normal U 2014;29(4):43-7.

[46] Zhang LL, Zhang WX. Personal future planning in middle and late adolescence and its relation to adolescents' communication with parents and friend. Acta Psychol Sinica 2008;40(5):583-92.

[47] Zhang WX, Xu FZ, Zhang LL, Wang SQ, Yu FJ, Gao T. The relationships of Chinese college students' personal future planning and attitude towards future with depression. Psychol Sci 2009;32(4):824-7.

[48] Creed PA, Wong OY, Hood M. Career decision-making, career barriers and occupational aspirations in Chinese adolescents. Int J Educ Vocat Guid 2009;9(3):189-203.

[49] Yates TM, Egeland B, Sroufe A. Rethinking resilience. In: Luthar SS, editor. Resilience and vulnerability: Adaptation in the context of childhood adversity. Cambridge: Cambridge University Press, 2003:243-66.

[50] Steinberg L, Graham S, O'Brien L, Woolard J, Cauffman E, Banich M. Age differences in future orientation and delay discounting. Child Dev 2009;80(1):28-44. doi: http://dx.doi.org/10.1111/j.1467-8624.2008.01244.x

[51] Gao SL, Chan KL. Future orientation and school bullying among adolescents in rural China: The mediating role of school bonding. Sage Open 2015;5(1):1-9.

[52] Nurmi JE. Age, sex, social class, and quality of family interaction as determinants of adolescents' future orientation: A developmental task interpretation. Adolescence 1987;22(88):977-91.

[53] Kerpelman JL, Mosher LS. Rural African American adolescents' future orientation: The importance of self-efficacy, control and responsibility, and identity development. Identity: Int J Theor Res 2004;4(2):187-208. doi: http://dx.doi.org/10.1207/s1532706xid0402_5.

[54] Kerpelman JL, Eryigit S, Stephens CJ. African American adolescents' future education orientation: Associations with self-efficacy, ethnic identity, and perceived parental support. J Youth Adolesc 2008;37(8):997-1008. doi: http://dx.doi.org/10.1007/s10964-007-9201-7.

[55] Zong JS, Li XP. Relationship between vocational students' characteristics of hope, self-esteem and career decision-making self-efficacy. J Southwest Jiaotong U 2014;15(5):84-8.

[56] Bandura A. Self-efficacy mechanism in human agency. Am Psychol 1982;37(2):122.

[57] Brooks RB. Children at risk: Fostering resilience and hope. Am J Orthopsychiatry 1994; 64(4):545-53.

[58] Gore J, Holmes K, Smith M, Southgate E, Albright J. Socioeconomic status and the career aspirations of Australian school students: Testing enduring assumptions. Aust Educ Res 2015;42(2):155-77.

[59] Jiang YJ. The status quo and features of poor college students' level of aspiration. J Henan Univ (Soc Sci) 2011;51(6):139-43.

[60] Neblett NG, Cortina KS. Adolescents' thoughts about parents' jobs and their importance for adolescents' future orientation. J Adolesc 2006;29:795-811.

[61] Trommsdorff G. Future orientation and socialization. Int J Psychol 1983;18(1-4):381-406.

[62] Ni H, Li C, Zhao J. Cultural consideration of resilience for Chinese immigrant children and adolescents. North Am J Med Sci 2014;7(3):112-6.

[63] Nurmi JE, Pulliainen H. The changing parent-child relationship, self-esteem, and intelligence as determinants of orientation to the future during early adolescence. J Adolesc 1991;14(1):35-51.

[64] Nurmi JE. How do adolescents see their future? A review of the development of future orientation and planning. Dev Rev 1991;11:1-59.

[65] Lekes N, Gingras I, Philippe FL, Koestner R, Fang J. Parental autonomy-support, intrinsic life goals, and well-being among adolescents in China and North America. J Youth Adolesc 2010;39(8):858-69.

[66] Wu WC, Chen DF. Research on the relationship between parenting style and college students' resilience. J Shaoguan U 2014;35(11):155-8.

[67] Benner AD, Mistry RS. Congruence of mother and teacher educational expectations and low-income youth's academic competence. J Educ Psychol 2007;99(1):140-53.

[68] Leong FTL, Serafica FC. Career development of Asian Americans: A research area in need of a good theory. In: Leong FTL, editor. Career development and vocational behavior of racial and ethnic minorities. New York: Lawrence Erlbaum, 1995:67-102.

[69] Fuligni AJ, Zhang W. Attitudes toward family obligation among adolescents in contemporary urban and rural China. Child Dev 2004;75(1):180-92.

[70] Leung SA, Chen PH. Counseling psychology in Chinese communities in Asia indigenous, multicultural, and cross-cultural considerations. Couns Psychol 2009;37(7):944-66.

[71] Chen P, Vazsonyi AT. Future orientation, school contexts, and problem behaviors: A multilevel study. J Youth Adolesc 2013;42(1):67-81.

[72] Crespo C, Jose PE, Kielpikowski M, Pryor J. "On solid ground": Family and school connectedness promotes adolescents' future orientation. J Adolesc 2013;36(5):993-1002. doi: http://dx.doi.org/10.1016/j.adolescence.2013.08.004.

[73] Coleman JC. The parenting of adolescents in Britain today. Child Soc 1997;11(1):44-52.

In: Soft Skills and Aspirations … ISBN: 978-1-53614-092-7
Editors: Daniel TL Shek, et al.

Chapter 8

DEVELOPMENTAL IMPACT OF DREAMS, ASPIRATIONS AND RELATED BEHAVIOR IN CHILDREN AND ADOLESCENTS

Florence KY Wu[1,*], EdD,
Daniel TL Shek[1-5], PhD, FHKPS, BBS, JP
and Hildie Leung[1], PhD
[1]Department of Applied Social Sciences,
The Hong Kong Polytechnic University, Hong Kong, PR China
[2]Centre for Innovative Programmes for Adolescents and Families,
The Hong Kong Polytechnic University, Hong Kong, PR China
[3]Department of Social Work, East China Normal University,
Shanghai, PR China
[4]Kiang Wu Nursing College of Macau, Macau, PR China
[5]Division of Adolescent Medicine, Kentucky Children's Hospital,
University of Kentucky College of Medicine,
Lexington, Kentucky, US

---

[*] Corresponding Author Email: florence.wu@polyu.edu.hk.

ABSTRACT

"Dreams," "aspirations" and related constructs are traditionally regarded as facilitators of adolescent educational attainment in the Chinese context. Besides, there is an emergent trend to widen the understanding of such constructs, particularly their impact on children and adolescent developmental outcomes. This chapter discusses the developmental outcomes of dreams, aspiration and related concepts based on a thorough review of the literature. Besides outlining the impacts of aspirations, dreams and related constructs on children and adolescents, features of related intervention programs, including themes of the intervention programs, program participants, methods of implementation and evaluation in both Western and Chinese contexts are also documented.

INTRODUCTION

In both Western and Chinese contexts, education has been increasingly perceived as the "vehicle for meritocracy and social mobility" (1). Nurturing children and adolescents with high educational attainment becomes the "mission" of education at all levels. However, numerous scholars cautioned that the increasing focus on educational attainment hinders the children and adolescents to aspire for their own genuine pursuit of future and adversely affects their physical and psychological health (2-4). Hence, it is of equal importance to encourage children and adolescents to boldly dream about their future in addition to educational attainment. Truitt et al. (5) encouraged adolescents to "dream high" so that high-hope children and adolescents would perceive the obstacles to goals as "temporary" and the high level of goal-directed motivation allows them to search for "the best alternative way." It is therefore fundamental to arouse the awareness of educators, parents and human service providers of the consequences of dreams and aspirations in children and how they can assist them to "aim for something higher" (1).

As mentioned in another paper in this special issue, a collaborative research named "iDream" was conducted (a) to understand the scientific underpinnings of instilling dreams, aspirations, hope, future orientation and related qualities in children and adolescents, (b) to investigate the positive impact of such constructs on children's and adolescents' well-being and overall development, and (c) to review existing interventions based on the related constructs with the financial support of the Bao Bao Bear Care Foundation Limited. The Bao Bao Bear Care Foundation Limited was founded in 2008 subsequent to the Sichuan earthquake to facilitate the provision of programs to children in Sichuan, China. The vision of the organization is that in spite of adverse experiences, children should not be deprived of the opportunity to experience a sense of hope. The iDream initiative was thus established to inspire and encourage children to explore their dreams and to promote their future orientation. It is believed that by exposing children to the success stories of various professionals, children would be able to understand the life trajectory leading to success and generate hope for their own future.

The chapter is based on the final report of the collaborative research (6) with a focus on three aspects of the study: (a) methodology of the literature review, (b) consequences of having dreams and aspirations, and (c) existing interventions on the promotion of dreams, aspirations and related psychology in children and adolescents.

OUR REVIEW

Conducting literature review is a process of "re-viewing" the existing literature to create a new dimension or fresh perspective to sharpen the conceptual understanding (7). Hart (8) reminded researchers that the need to thoroughly understand the body of knowledge is crucial before administering any research. According to Pawson and his colleagues (9), there are seven steps for a systematic review, namely: 1) clarify the scope of review; 2) search for relevant evidence; 3) appraise quality of studies using judgment to supplement formal checklists; 4) extract different data from different studies; 5) synthesize data to achieve refinement of the literature; 6) make recommendations; and 7) disseminate findings and evaluate the extent to which the findings are able to benefit the field.

In the present literature review, the scope is about the dreams, aspirations and related development in children and adolescents. Besides, the features of effective intervention programs in these areas in the context of China would be described. The peer-reviewed literature search methodology was adopted to re-view the literature related to hope and dreams of children and adolescents and a quasi-realist approach (9) was utilized to synthesize the data with reference to (a) conceptual review of the concepts covered in the present literature review; (b) antecedents affecting the development of hope and aspirations of children and adolescents; and (c) possible outcomes of having developed the attributes. According to Pawson et al. (9), the quasi-realist approach has been frequently utilized to generate reliable and usable findings for describing how complex interventions function in different contexts. This approach is not over-relying upon the review of "what works" but yielding the understanding of what works "for whom, under what circumstances, in what respects and how" (9). This requires moving beyond typical study design assessment criteria such as statistical power and sampling design. The focus lies on the descriptive details about the intervention process and context instead. The "quasi-" approach helps to look into the different population orientations and multi-level components that would help substantiate the understanding of what effective and appropriate programs could be implemented in China.

Peer-Reviewed Literature Search Methodology

To identify relevant literature for the review, a detailed search of the literature published during the period between 1980 and 2015 was conducted from February to June, 2015, with the use of the online databases, including PsycINFO, Academic Search Premier, Web of Science, EBSCOhost database and China's database CAJ Full-text Database. CAJ Full-text Database was adopted for searching articles published in China. The single keyword "dreams," "hope," "aspirations," "future orientation," "resilience," "beliefs in the future," "children," "adolescents" and the combinations of keywords with Boolean operators (and/or/*) were utilized as the search (e.g., "dreams AND hope AND children"; "aspirations AND future orientation"; "hope" OR "aspirations"; "child* AND adolescents*"; "China OR Chinese OR Hong Kong*"). Articles were included if they met the following four selection criteria: 1) the focus is on youth population which was defined a prior as individuals aged between 6 and 18 years; 2) the study or program addressed the conceptualization of dream or related concepts; 3) the study or program covered the development or validation of measurement tools of dreams or its related concepts and 4) the study or program was conducted or developed either in the Chinese or Western context.

The initial focus of the review was on Western and China-based research, with special focus on the context of China. All articles in English and Chinese were included, as were articles in other languages in which an English or Chinese abstract was available. The titles of all publications were identified with possible relevance. The abstracts were reviewed if they appeared to meet the selection criteria. The full publication would then be obtained and decision was made whether the article should be included or not. There were altogether 223 articles, with 144 being found in the international databases and 79 in China's database.

In order to produce reliable and comparable findings from the existing literature and to decide if the knowledge obtained could be translated into new directions and interventions, there is an immense need to adopt a systematic approach to "appraise, interpret and synthesize literature from divert source" (10). The systematic approach requires a set of clear arguments to review and synthesize the literature. Therefore, the quasi-realist approach was adopted to gauge the understanding of "what really works" for the children and adolescents in developing hope and aspirations and of other knowledge beyond this understanding.

CONSEQUENCES OF DREAMS, ASPIRATIONS AND RELATED DEVELOPMENT

The present literature review suggests that dream and its related constructs such as resilience, hope, aspirations, future orientation, and belief in the future are positively associated with children and adolescent outcomes across different domains, including the psychological, academic, vocational, and behavioral domains.

Psychological outcomes

The positive impact of resilience, hope, and aspirations on children's and adolescents' psychological well-being is well documented in the Western literature. More hopeful adolescents reported higher levels of life satisfaction (4, 11-14) and lower levels of psychological distress (11). Hope also acted as a buffer against the impact of negative or stressful life events on life satisfaction (4). Similarly, adolescents with more positive beliefs in the future possessed higher self-esteem and self-efficacy (15). More resilient youths also perceived lower levels of stress and were more satisfied with life (16).

The majority of the studies conducted in China focused on examining the impact of resilience and aspirations on psychological well-being of children and adolescents, especially those who experienced negative life events (e.g., survivors of earthquakes, children of parents with HIV). Findings are consistent with the Western literature that resilient youths experienced higher levels of life satisfaction (17) and were less likely to demonstrate obsessive-compulsive (18), depressive (19, 20), and post-traumatic stress disorder symptoms (21). Future orientation also predicted Chinese adolescents' levels of anxiety, depression (22) and subjective well-being. The positive impact of resilience, hope, and future orientation on individual's psychological well-being may be explained by several factors: 1) resilient children and adolescents often experience higher levels of positive emotions than their less resilient counterparts, even in times of difficulties; 2) they are able to use cognitive coping strategies such as finding opportunities for growth from challenges; 3) it is believed that they have the ability to control their environment; and 4) they set realistic goals which may help them reduce difficulties in life (16).

Lastly, Gan et al. (23) found that positive future expectations were significantly correlated with resilience among adolescents who experienced the Sichuan earthquake. Indeed, the findings point toward the fact that less resilient adolescents may have difficulty in envisioning or thinking positively about their future and that "a person's future is not merely the result of his or her life circumstances; the future is also predicted by the manner in which a person thinks about it" (23). The findings have important implications for the integration of both resilience and future expectation components in interventions.

Academic outcomes

Evidence from studies in the West generally showed that adolescents with higher levels of future orientation had higher academic achievement (24). They attached significantly higher value to achievement of academic goals and perceived studying hard as instrumental in achieving goals (25). Similarly, more hopeful youths tend to have higher academic achievement (12, 26, 27) as well. Many studies on the impact of students' aspirations on academic achievement showed similar observations, where students with higher levels of aspirations showed higher levels of Grade Point Averages (28, 29) and increased school engagement across domains including behavioral, emotional, and cognitive engagement (29). In a longitudinal study of the impact of adolescent future orientation on adult educational attainment, Beal and Crockett (30) also found that adolescent aspirations positively predicted adult educational attainment eight years later. Similarly, future orientation increased students' likelihood of staying in school (31) and attending college (32).

Similar findings were observed in studies conducted in China. Zhao and colleagues (33) examined correlates of problem behaviors among children affected by HIV and found that low educational aspirations had direct negative effects on school adjustment. Children's early expectations were strong predictors of children's chances of staying in school, completing compulsory education and completing secondary education as well (34).

Zhang (34) found that future orientation had positive influences on junior secondary school students' learning attitude, academic help-seeking behavior and academic achievement. Chen (35) also found that university students who were more future-oriented were more engaged in their studies. Higher levels of resilience were also associated with better educational outcomes of migrant children, including more effort put into study, higher educational aspirations, and less intention to drop out of school (36).

The positive associations between aspiration-related variables and academic outcomes may be due to several factors. First, adolescents with high aspirations develop goals for the future, which serves as a motivation for higher academic achievement. Second, high-hope students are more willing to find solutions when they encounter difficulties and try new approaches. On the other hand, low-hope students are often more passive and seldom learn from past experiences, which may hinder academic achievement. As pointed out by Snyder et al. (27), "teaching hopeful thinking has the potential to improve the students' goal pursuits in all areas of their lives, thereby leading to more positive emotions, greater psychological adjustment, and more social support" (27).

Vocational outcomes

In terms of career related outcomes, studies from the West generally showed that adolescents with higher levels of aspirations had higher levels of future career accomplishments and achievement (37-42). For instance, in a longitudinal study in the United Kingdom, Schoon and Polek (43) found that career aspirations measured at age 16 years positively predicted career attainment in their mid-30s, even after controlling family background and cognitive ability. Specifically, teens who aspired to a professional job were more likely to pursue further education and were more likely to achieve their occupational aspirations as adults. Few studies were directly related to the variables of interest in the context of China, with some exceptions of scholars examining the impact of occupational expectations on vocational outcomes. It was reasoned that more hopeful and highly aspired youths may be more persistent and ambitious to achieve their career goals (43). For instance, Huang and Bashir (44) found that occupational expectations positively predicted occupational self-efficacy.

Strauss, Griffin and Parker (45) identified positive impact of "Future work self" on proactive career behavior. Although the study was conducted on postgraduate students, the findings yielded practical implications for youth hope-based interventions. A "Future work self" refers to "an individual's representation of himself or herself in the future that reflects his or her hopes and aspirations in relation to work. The clearer and more accessible this representation is, the more salient the Future work self is" (45). Individuals with a salient Future work self (i.e., they have a clear image of themselves in a future career) are more willing to take risks and set ambitious goals. They would broaden their creative thinking about future possibilities which motivate them to proactively shape their careers. These findings highlight the importance of cultivating elaborative Future work selves through career counseling. Role models may be used to help construct ideals and possible Future work selves. Cognitive strategies may also be taught to help students envision their Future work self.

Behavioral outcomes

Studies in both the Western and Chinese contexts showed that aspirations and related constructs serve as protective factors against the development of problem behaviors in children and adolescents. According to Robbins and Bryan (46), adolescents with stronger future orientation were more likely to perceive risk behaviors negatively. They were less likely to smoke cigarettes, use marijuana or hard drugs, or engage in problematic drinking (46-51). Regarding hope, Hagen and colleagues (52) found that more hopeful adolescents reported fewer internalizing and externalizing problems. In a longitudinal study of high school students, Ciarrochi and colleagues (26) reported that lower levels of hope predicted higher rates of behavioral problems (e.g., aggression, inattention). Hope was also related to lower levels of involvement in violence (53). Regarding the impact of aspiration on adolescent problem behaviors, most studies reported a negative relationship. Generally speaking, youths with high aspirations are less likely to drink alcohol or get drunk (54-57). They also reported lower levels of cigarette (54) and substance use (58), risky sexual behavior (59) and premarital child-bearing (60-64).

Compared to the West, few studies have been conducted to examine the impact of aspiration-related factors on problem behaviors among children and adolescents in China. Among the sparse articles identified, findings comparable to those reported in the West were found. For instance, Zhao and colleagues (33) found that low levels of educational aspiration were negatively associated with problem behaviors among orphans and vulnerable children affected by parental HIV. Li et al. (65) also found that middle school male students with lower educational expectations reported more cigarette smoking. Du et al. (66) conducted a study on rural-to-urban migrant children and found that individualistic orientation predicted higher levels of hopelessness and subsequently more substance use behavior. The authors reasoned that China is a collectivistic culture and thus collectivistic orientation (as opposed to individualism) and coping such as family support play important protective roles in developing hope and against engagement in problem behavior.

Besides problem behavior, some studies showed that aspiration-related constructs were correlated with healthy behaviors. For instance, youths who had a more positive belief about their ability to live a healthy lifestyle had better attitudes and skills in living a healthy lifestyle (e.g., exercising, eating healthily) (67). Highly aspired students were also more responsible for their health, and reported higher levels of nutrition and exercise (68). These findings underscore the important role of cognitive beliefs on attitudes and choices in lifestyle and health promoting behaviors. In terms of prosocial behaviors, Syvertsen et al. (69) found that rates of community service for youth with college aspirations increased considerably more than the rates of community service for those with other post-high school plans. Wang et al. (68) argued that adolescents who have higher levels of aspirations would be more likely to be prosocially involved in the community.

Taken as a whole, findings in both the Western and Chinese contexts showed the positive impact of hope, resilience, future orientation, beliefs in the future, and aspirations on different domains of children and adolescents' life, including the psychological, academic, vocational and behavioral domains. Findings highlight the importance of developing interventions that target both skill-building and efficacy-enhancing elements to help children and adolescents better understand their cognitive-affective responses to adversities, and providing them with the ability to take advantage of life opportunities to maintain a hopeful outlook on life.

EXISTING INTERVENTIONS

The literature review showed that there are many intervention programs implemented in the Western context to help children and adolescents to search for their dreams, hope and aspirations. Indeed, hope-based interventions that help students to explore their goals and identify actions to achieve have been shown to promote life satisfaction in students (12). In contrast, there are very limited intervention programs facilitating children and the youth to explore their dreams, aspirations and hopes in different Chinese contexts. In the past three decades, there were less than ten published intervention programs addressing aspiration and related constructs in China. Themes like exploring hope, future orientation or dreams for children and adolescents were scarcely found in the literature. As such, there is much capacity to develop intervention programs with these themes to help children and adolescents to understand themselves and capacities to realize their potential in mainland China.

Themes/foci of the intervention programs

The coverage of themes of the intervention programs implemented in the Western context is wide. For example, there are programs encouraging low-income youth or juvenile delinquents to explore the meaning of hope to them and what future orientation could be focused on if they wish to step out from their present situation (70, 71). There are also programs helping children of divorced families or adolescents with depression to strengthen their decision-making ability and thus developing their sense of self-efficacy and resilience (72-74). The intervention programs were designed for targeted children and the youth, and the contents were context- and target-group-specific. However, there are very few programs helping children or youth to explore their needs and aspirations.

Among the limited intervention programs in the Chinese context, "aspiration" is the major theme, with special attention to explore and develop "academic aspiration" of children and adolescents (75). There is a strong conviction that children's future is constituted by academic excellence in traditional Chinese context. Nurturing academic aspiration became the prime concern of the intervention programs in China and there are very few intervention programs exploring hope, aspiration or other aspects of future orientation. One interesting finding in the Western literature is that some of the program designers held quite strong beliefs about youth's educational or academic development, which aligned with the Chinese context, to help them understand what hope and aspiration mean to them (71, 76). They believed that creating successful academic experiences may help the youth to aspire to achieve ambitious goals later in life. However, the meaning of "success" or "aspiration" could be varied in youth's perspective with different cultural backgrounds. As such, there is an immense need to develop programs to help children and adolescents widen their exploration of their future hope or aspirations with their internal frame of reference in the Chinese context.

In Hong Kong, a successful positive youth development program entitled Project P.A.T.H.S. (denoting Positive Adolescent Training through Holistic Social Programmes) was developed and implemented for young adolescents in secondary schools (77-79). The program was intended to promote students' holistic development by enhancing their intrapersonal and interpersonal competencies. With particular relevance to the present review, the P.A.T.H.S. curriculum includes sessions aiming at promoting students' resilience, beliefs in the future, and spirituality for Secondary 1 to 3 students.

Indeed, most existing dream- and aspiration-based interventions in Chinese contexts focus on nurturing students' academic aspirations, which is merely one aspect of aspirations. However, the present review revealed that dreams and aspirations are far more encompassing. Therefore, it is important to encourage youngsters to discover their unique strengths and potential beyond merely academic achievements to reflect on and understand what interests them and what their meaning in life is. Moreover, it is important to equip adolescents with competencies such as resilience and help them adopt a positive outlook on life so that they are able to overcome adversities and challenges as they strive to achieve their dreams.

Program participants

Quite a number of intervention programs implemented in the Western contexts were designed for youths with special needs, such as low-income youth (71, 80), juvenile delinquents (70), AIDS-orphaned youths (81), children from single-parent families (76, 82) or children and adolescents with emotional and behavioral problems (83). The number of children and adolescents served in these programs varied from a few dozen youth (70, 84) to a few hundred children and adolescents from various schools (73, 85). Most of these programs had positive effects on the future orientation of the adolescents and they assisted young people to develop higher levels of continuity, hope and career decidedness. However, the abovementioned programs catered for specific target group of children and adolescents and there are limited programs helping youths in the general population to explore their dreams, aspirations or future orientation. Pittman and Irby (86) stated that "problem-free is not fully prepared." Hence, it is recommended to advocate programs catering for all the children and adolescents to allow them to experience the "exploration" and "creation" of their own dreams and aspirations.

In the context of China, the programs implemented have made an attempt to cater for youths in the general population without much restriction in the recruitment. However, the number of children and adolescents served was limited to a few dozens and the served participants were from the well-off cities, such as Beijing and Shanghai (75). There were few programs implemented to serve the children and adolescents in other provinces, especially the more rural villages or the remote western part of China. Lai (87) stated that the remote western region of China should actively prepare for the future development to reduce regional inequality that might hinder the future development of the children and adolescents in those areas. There is a need to extend the implementation of the interventions to these regions or provinces so that children and adolescents in these regions are able to be exposed to the development of the well-off regions. Most importantly, the future development of their regions will allow them to explore their own meanings of dreams, aspirations and future orientation with more understanding of the strengths and limitations of their own living environments.

With reference to the CEDAR (Career Exploration, Development, and Resources group) program, the Chinese youths who newly immigrated to the United States struggled with language barriers, cultural adjustment and academic demands and many of them expressed "uncertainty about their future" (88). The "uncertainty" is applicable to the mainland Chinese adolescents as well. Yong people might have followed their families to move to different provinces as migrant children or adolescents. The migrant adolescents found it difficult to adapt to school or other social settings. When programs are designed for the mainland children and adolescents to explore their future aspirations or dreams, these difficulties should be well aware of and acknowledged. Hence a trustworthy and open atmosphere could be cultivated in the programs in which the adolescents could share their values and discuss challenges they would perceive as barriers in the environment.

Methods of implementation

In the Western contexts, the intervention approach varied from intensive arranged activities, such as summer camps (85) or intensive classes arranged every school day for three months (70), to class-based or curriculum-based lessons held regularly with interactive activities (84, 89, 90). For the intensive programs, the participants reported significant changes of having more ability to initiate and sustain movement toward their goals and having the ability to create positive future for themselves right after participating the programs. However, the researchers expressed their concern over the sustainability of these changes on children and adolescents since there were few longitudinal follow-up studies to show long-lasting effects on the participants (85).

For the class-based or curriculum-based intervention programs, the participants reported positive effects on developing goals and aspirations and having higher levels of hope and optimism. There are positive long-term effects on the participants in these programs as the participants were given sufficient time to incorporate the training and learning in the programs with their life experiences (71, 81). The regularly-held classes (either incorporated into school curriculum or arranged as after-school programs) provided a steady time-frame to the youth participants to learn regularly and gradually, creating a stable social-friendly environment to the participants to establish social connection with other participants.

Some intervention programs carried out in the Western contexts were individual-based such as individual psychotherapy session (91) or in-home sessions (74). The participants served in these programs were quite limited (8 to 15 participants) of targeted youth population. Besides, the small-scale designs did not instill significant positive changes in the participants in understanding hope and generating aspirations (74).

In the context of China, mere lecturing and collective instructions are the most common approaches in helping children and adolescents to understand what "aspirations," "dreams" or "future orientation" means in these programs (92, 93). The teachers or facilitators of the programs taught what "aspirations" or "future goals" were and students learned the concepts in a more directive and guided manner. There is rare opportunity for children and adolescents to explore the meanings of "aspirations," "hopes" or "dreams" to themselves in class. Even though some implementers arranged outdoor activities such as visits to museums of traditional Chinese heroes (75), interactive classroom activities (including group discussions, role-plays or card games) or engaging teaching approaches (including self-disclosure of teachers and students or collaborative learning) were seldom carried out in these programs. Interactive classroom activities and engaging teaching approaches were found effective in assisting adolescents to look inwardly upon their genuine needs and producing better implementation quality in the Chinese context (94). Some programs have adopted the group counseling approach to assist the Chinese immigrant youth in the United States to explore their career interests, skills, abilities, priorities and different career options (95). The group counseling approach is able to provide a "safe haven" for the Chinese youth participants to share their concerns and aspirations in a trustworthy milieu and the collaboration. The communication among the participants helps weave the friendship web that provides socio-emotional support and great resources to the participants. Incorporating these approaches into the intervention programs in the context of China might help facilitate the children and adolescents to search for their own meanings of aspirations, hopes and dreams instead of being taught by the teachers or implementers.

Practical information such as college applications or resume writing has also been provided in some of the programs and the information provided has helped the participants foster a sense of competence in career exploration (88, 95). However, the provision of hands-on information on the work lives of different professionals is rarely found in the literature, especially in the Chinese context. It is recommended to prepare more hands-on information for the participants, for example introducing the work values, ethics or prospect of different professionals, or resume writing and college applications.

Besides approaches and intervention methods, implementers in the intervention programs also varied. The implementers of intervention programs in the Western contexts are mostly professionals in human service such as educationalists, psychologists, counselors, social workers or researchers of the programs. For example, the programs helping the low-income youth and aiming to reduce their hopelessness invited school personnel (teachers or guidance counselors) or career counseling psychologist to deliver the programs (72, 73). In addition to these professionals in human services, other professionals such as professional dancers or artists were also invited as collaborators (80, 85). The professionalism of the implementers helped deliver professional knowledge to the participants and thus enriched the participants' understanding of the related concepts. The involvement of the implementers other than human service professionals exposed the participants to new leisure or career options and opportunities (70). However, the professional image of the implementers has distanced the participants and might have hindered the engagement between the implementers and the participants. More preparation work, such as pre-program meetings with the participants or extra time offered to the participants to know the implementers in each session, has to be done when involving professional counterparts in the intervention programs.

Chung (96) observed that Asian clients have a tendency to expect directive guidance, information-driven and problem-solving approach to assist them for the personal and career exploration. That is why the Chinese participants of these intervention programs would have high expectations on the facilitators to serve multiple roles such as an adviser, a role model, an authority to provide directions, and an expert with solid professional knowledge. The implementers would use different means to facilitate the participants to explore and search for their potential and aspirations in an in-depth manner by, for example, arranging the students or participants in groups, using card games, discussions, and reflective exercises. Some of the implementers have utilized the imitating case scenarios for small group discussion (95). Making use of the case scenarios was less intimidating and was more congruent with Chinese concern with "loss of face" in disclosing their thoughts, wishes, perceived "unrealistic" dreams (that might be their genuine dreams) and feelings toward achieving these dreams and wishes (97).

One of the unique features of the intervention programs in both Western and Chinese contexts is to invite guest speakers, such as alumni or professionals from different fields (70, 78, 95), to share 1) their experiences of how they chose their career pathways; 2) struggles met in the process and 3) ways to be resilient in facing obstacles. Some of the guest speakers shared similar backgrounds of the participants (e.g., the alumni) to draw closer linkages to the children or adolescent participants (70) and some of the guest speakers were the successful figures in the society to arouse participants' interests to better understand the respective field. In the 1980s, the focus of sharing was about how to set goals and their success stories (75). The guest speakers typically acted like the "role models" for the participants to demonstrate the possibilities of being competent in respective fields. The feasible "accessibility" to these significant others in the participants' socio-cultural system offers prime opportunities for the youth to explore more educational and vocational possibilities, ways to pursue their aspirations and hopes, as well as the basic or fundamental skills in respective workplaces (54, 95).

Some final remarks on evaluation are in order. Different methods have been used to evaluate the programs under review. A number of programs have shown the effectiveness in helping their participants to reduce their sense of hopelessness (72), increase adolescents' hope for the future (73, 80, 85), occupational, educational and academic aspiration (79) and enhance resilience of children and adolescents (89, 98). However, there are very few longitudinal evaluation studies to investigate the long-term impacts of these programs on the participants. The importance of administering longitudinal studies is shown in some pioneering positive youth development programs in the Chinese context (99). Administering program evaluation is crucial to understand "how" and "why" the program works (100).

CONCLUSION

In this review, we examined the consequences of having dreams, aspirations and related attributes. Studies have shown that resilience, aspirations, and future orientation serve as protective factors against problem behaviors. Students with lower levels of future orientation were more likely to engage in problem behaviors such as smoking, drinking, or drug abuse. Moreover, high school students with low levels of hope exhibited more externalizing behaviors (e.g., aggression, delinquency). In addition, positive youth development studies have also shown that resilient youths, who had a positive belief in the future and/or a higher level of spirituality (including a meaning and purpose in life), reported higher levels of connectedness to the community and a sense of contribution, which serves as protective factors against the development of problem behaviors.

The present study also documented features of the intervention programs implemented in both Western and Chinese contexts. It is recommended to design and implement indigenous intervention programs that meet the needs of Chinese children and adolescents in the context of China. The specific Chinese culture has been quite often overlooked in implementing intervention programs on aspirations, hope or resilience building. Leong and Gim-Chung (101) cautioned that the submissive and passive image drawn by traditional patriarchal society might confine the range of exploration and choices of Chinese adolescents (especially female youths) when they make life-long decisions. Hence, program implementers have to be well aware of these subtle Chinese cultural concerns while they are carrying out intervention programs. In particular, it is crucial to create an open and trustworthy environment for the youth participants to process personal yet complex feelings and thoughts during the process of program implementation.

ACKNOWLEDGMENTS

The current project was financially supported by The Bao Bao Bear Care Foundation Limited. The materials in this paper are based on a paper published in the *International Journal on Disability and Human Development* 2017;16(4) issue.

REFERENCES

[1] Rose J, Baird JA. Aspirations and an austerity state: Young people's hopes and goals for the future. London Rev Educ 2013;11(2):157-73.

[2] Juvakka T, Kylmä J. Hope in adolescents with cancer. Eur J Oncol Nurs 2009;13(3):193-9.

[3] Spohrer K. Deconstructing 'Aspiration': UK policy debates and European policy trends. Educ Res Eval 2011;10(1):53-63.

[4] Valle MF, Huebner ES, Suldo SM. An analysis of hope as a psychological strength. J Sch Psychol 2006;44(5):393-406.

[5] Truitt M, Biesecker B, Capone G, Bailey T, Erby L. The role of hope in adaptation to uncertainty: The experience of caregivers of children with Down syndrome. Patient Educ Couns 2012; 87:233-8.

[6] Wu FK, Leung H, Shek DTL. Collaborative research report on "Literature review on hope and aspirations in children and adolescents." [Unpublished manuscript] Hong Kong: Department of Applied Social Sciences, The Hong Kong Polytechnic University, 2015.

[7] Jesson J, Matheson L, Lacey FM. Doing your literature review: Traditional and systematic techniques. London: Sage, 2011.

[8] Hart C. Doing a literature review: Releasing the social science research imagination. London: Sage, 1998.

[9] Pawson R, Greenhalgh T, Harvey G, Walshe K. Realist synthesis: An introduction. Manchester: ESRC Research Methods Programme, University of Manchester, 2004.

[10] Khanlou N, Wray R. A whole community approach toward child and youth resilience promotion: A review of resilience literature. Int J Ment Health Addict 2014;12(1):64-79.

[11] Gilman R, Dooley J, Florell D. Relative levels of hope and their relationship with academic and psychological indicators among adolescents. J Soc Clin Psychol 2006;25(2):166-78.

[12] Marques SC, Pais-Ribeiro JL, Lopez SJ. The role of positive psychology constructs in predicting mental health and academic achievement in children and adolescents: A two-year longitudinal study. J Happiness Stud 2011;12(6):1049-62.

[13] Marques SC, Lopez SJ, Mitchell J. The role of hope, spirituality and religious practice in adolescents' life satisfaction: Longitudinal findings. J Happiness Stud 2013;14(1):251-61.

[14] Vacek KR, Coyle LD, Vera EM. Stress, self-Esteem, hope, optimism, and well-being in urban, ethnic minority adolescents. J Multicult Couns Devel 2010;38(2):99-111.

[15] Bryan A, Aiken LS, West SG. HIV/STD risk among incarcerated adolescents: Optimism about the future and self-esteem as predictors of condom use self-efficacy. J Appl Soc Psychol 2004;34(5):912-36.

[16] Abolghasemi A, Varaniyab ST. Resilience and perceived stress: Predictors of life satisfaction in the students of success and failure. Procedia Soc Behav Sci 2010; 5:748-52.

[17] Liu Y, Wang ZH, Li ZG. Affective mediators of the influence of neuroticism and resilience on life satisfaction. Pers Individ Dif 2012;52(7):833-8.

[18] Sun J, Li ZJ, Buys NJ, Storch EA, Wang JS. Obsessive-compulsive symptoms and personal disposition, family coherence and school environment in Chinese adolescents: A resilience approach. J Affect Disord 2014; 168:459-65.

[19] Wang B, Li X, Barnett D, Zhao G, Zhao J, Stanton B. Risk and protective factors for depression symptoms among children affected by HIV/AIDS in rural China: A structural equation modeling analysis. Soc Sci Med 2012;74(9):1435-43.

[20] Ye Y, Fan F, Li L, Han Q. Trajectory and predictors of depressive symptoms among adolescent survivors following the Wenchuan earthquake in China: A cohort study. Soc Psychiatry Psychiatr Epidemiol 2014;49(6):943-52.

[21] Ying L, Wu X, Lin C, Jiang L. Traumatic severity and trait resilience as predictors of posttraumatic stress disorder and depressive symptoms among adolescent survivors of the Wenchuan earthquake. PLoS One 2014;9(2):e89401.

[22] Yu XN, Lau JTF, Mak WWS, Zhang J, Lui WWF, Zhang J. Factor structure and psychometric properties of the Connor-Davidson Resilience Scale among Chinese adolescents. Compr Psychiatry 2011;52(2):218-24.

[23] Gan Y, Xie X, Wang T, Rodriguez MA, Tang CS. Thriving in the shadow of the 2008 Sichuan earthquake: Two studies on resilience in adolescents. J Health Psychol 2013;18(9):1232-41.

[24] Mello ZR, Worrell FC. The relationship of time perspective to age, gender, and academic achievement among academically talented adolescents. J Educ Gifted 2006;29(3):271-89.

[25] De Volder ML, Lens W. Academic achievement and future time perspective as a cognitive-motivational concept. J Pers Soc Psychol 1982;42(3):566-71.

[26] Ciarrochi J, Heaven PC, Davies F. The impact of hope, self-esteem, and attributional style on adolescents‘ school grades and emotional well-being: A longitudinal study. J Res Pers 2007;41(6):1161-78.

[27] Snyder CR, Shorey HS, Cheavens J, Pulvers KM, Adams III VH, Wiklund C. Hope and academic success in college. J Educ Psychol 2002;94(4):820-6.

[28] Akos P, Lambie G, Milsom A, Gilbert K. Early adolescents‘ aspirations and academic tracking: An exploratory investigation. Sch Couns 2007;11(1):57-64.

[29] Hill NE, Wang MT. From middle school to college: Developing aspirations, promoting engagement, and indirect pathways from parenting to post high school enrollment. Dev Psychol 2015;51(2):224-35.

[30] Beal SJ, Crockett LJ. Adolescents' occupational and educational aspirations and expectations: Links to high school activities and adult educational attainment. Dev Psychol 2010;46(1):258-65.

[31] Marjoribanks K. Family contexts, individual characteristics, proximal settings, and adolescents‘ aspirations. Psychol Rep 2002;91:769-79.

[32] South SJ, Baumer EP, Lutz A. Interpreting community effects on youth educational attainment. Youth Soc 2003;35(1):3-36.

[33] Zhao Q, Li X, Gu C, Zhao J, Zhao G. Correlates and mediators of problem behaviors among children affected by HIV/AIDS in rural China: A structural equation modeling analysis. J Child Fam Stud 2014:1-13.

[34] Zhang Y. The hopes carry them on: Early educational expectations and later educational outcomes in rural Gansu, China. In: Kao R, Park H, eds. Family

[35] Environments, School Resources, and Educational Outcomes. Chen Y. The relationship of university students' future orientation, specialty identity and study engagement. Sichuan U Arts Sci J 2013;23(2):91-5.

[36] Wu Q, Tsang B, Ming H. Social capital, family support, resilience and educational outcomes of Chinese migrant children. Br J Soc Work 2014;44(3):636-56.

[37] Cochran DB, Wang EW, Stevenson SJ, Johnson LE, Crews C. Adolescent occupational aspirations: Test of Gottfredson's theory of circumscription and compromise. Career Dev Q 2011;59(5):412-27.

[38] Croll P. Occupational choice, socio-economic status and educational attainment: A study of the occupational choices and destinations of young people in the British Household Panel Survey. Res Papers in Educ 2008;23(3):243-68.

[39] Marjoribanks K. Family learning environments and students' outcomes: A review. J Comp Fam Stud 1996:373-94.

[40] Schoon I, Martin P, Ross A. Career transitions in times of social change. His and her story. J Vocat Behav 2007;70(1):78-96.

[41] Schoon I, Parsons S. Teenage aspirations for future careers and occupational outcomes. J Vocat Behav 2002;60(2):262-88.

[42] Yates S, Harris A, Sabates R, Staff J. Early occupational aspirations and fractured transitions: A study of entry into 'NEET' status in the UK. J Soc Policy 2011;40(3):513-34.

[43] Schoon I, Polek E. Teenage career aspirations and adult career attainment: The role of gender, social background and general cognitive ability. Int J Behav Dev 2011;35(3):210-7.

[44] Huang HY, Bashir M. Examining the gender gap in information assurance: A study of psychological factors. In HCI International 2015-Posters' Extended Abstracts. Springer International Publishing, 2015:117-22.

[45] Strauss K, Griffin MA, Parker SK. Future work selves: How salient hoped-for identities motivate proactive career behaviors. J Appl Psychol 2012;97(3):580-98.

[46] Robbins RN, Bryan A. Relationships between future orientation, impulsive sensation seeking, and risk behavior among adjudicated adolescents. J Adolesc Res 2004;19(4):428-45.

[47] Adams J. Consideration of immediate and future consequences, smoking status, and body mass index. Health Psychol 2012;31(2):260.

[48] Barnett E, Spruijt-Metz D, Unger JB, Rohrbach LA, Sun P, Sussman S. Bidirectional associations between future time perspective and substance use among continuation high-school students. Subst Use Misuse 2013;48(8):574-80.

[49] Chen P, Vazsonyi AT. Future orientation, school contexts, and problem behaviors: A multilevel study. J Youth Adolesc 2013;42(1):67-81.
[50] McCay BJ, Jones PJ. Marine protected areas and the governance of marine ecosystems and fisheries. Conserv Biol 2011;25(6):1130-3.
[51] Peters RJ, Tortolero SR, Johnson RJ, Addy RC, Markham CM, Escobar-Chaves SL, et al. The relationship between future orientation and street substance use among Texas alternative school students. Am J Addict 2005;14(5):478-85.
[52] Hagen KA, Myers BJ, Mackintosh VH. Hope, social support, and behavioral problems in at-risk children. Am J Orthopsychiatry 2005;75(2):211-9.
[53] Stoddard SA, McMorris BJ, Sieving RE. Do social connections and hope matter in predicting early adolescent violence? Am J Community Psychol 2011;48(3-4):247-56.
[54] Cook WK, Hofstetter CR, Kang M, Hovell MF, Irvin V. Rethinking acculturation: A study of alcohol use of Korean American adolescents in Southern California. Contemp Drug Probl 2009;36(1-2):217.
[55] Crum RM, Storr CL, Anthony JC. Are educational aspirations associated with the risk of alcohol use and alcohol use-related problems among adolescents? Subst Use Misuse 2005;40(2):151-69.
[56] Dunn MS, Kitts C, Lewis S, Goodrow B, Scherzer GD. Effects of youth assets on adolescent alcohol, tobacco, marijuana use, and sexual behavior. J Alcohol Drug Educ 2011;55(3):23-40.
[57] Liu XC, Keyes KM, Li G. Work stress and alcohol consumption among adolescents: Moderation by family and peer influences. BMC Public Health 2014;14(1):1303.
[58] Henry KL. Who's skipping school: Characteristics of truants in 8th and 10th grade. J Sch Health 2007;77(1):29-35.
[59] Kalina O, Geckova AM, Klein D, Jarcuska P, Orosova O, van Dijk JP, et al. Psychosocial factors associated with sexual behaviour in early adolescence. Eur J Contracept Reprod Health Care 2011;16(4):298-306.
[60] Davis TM. An examination of repeat pregnancies using problem behavior theory: Is it really problematic? J Youth Stud 2002;5(3):337-51.
[61] East PL. Racial and ethnic differences in girls' sexual, marital, and birth expectations. J Marriage Fam 1998;60(1):150-62.
[62] O'Connor ML. Academically oriented teenage women have reduced pregnancy risk. Perspect Sex Reprod Health 1999;31(2):105-6.
[63] Plotnick RD. The effects of attitudes on teenage premarital pregnancy and its resolution. Am Sociol Rev 1992;57(6):800-11.
[64] Witwer M. Pregnancy risk lessened for teenagers with high educational aspirations. Perspect Sex Reprod Health 1993;25(4):189.
[65] Li X, Fang X, Stanton B. Cigarette smoking among schoolboys in Beijing, China. J Adolesc 1999;22(5):621-5.

[66] Du H, Li X, Lin D, Tam CC. Hopelessness, individualism, collectivism, and substance use among young rural-to-urban migrants in China. Health Psychol Behav Med 2014;2(1):211-20.

[67] Kelly SA, Melnyk BM, Jacobson DL, O'Haver JA. Correlates among healthy lifestyle cognitive beliefs, healthy lifestyle choices, social support, and healthy behaviors in adolescents: Implications for behavioral change strategies and future research. J Pediatr Health Care 2011;25(4):216-23.

[68] Wang RH, Chen SW, Tang SM, Lee SL, Jian SY. The relationship between selected developmental assets and health-promoting behaviours of adolescents in Southern Taiwan. J Clin Nurs 2011;20(3-4):359-68.

[69] Syvertsen AK, Wray-Lake L, Flanagan CA, Wayne Osgood D, Briddell L. Thirty-year trends in US adolescents' civic engagement: A story of changing participation and educational differences. J Res Adolesc 2011;21(3):586-94.

[70] Carruthers C. Processes and outcomes of an after-school program for adolescent girls. J Park Recreat Admi 2006;24(4).

[71] Purtell KM, McLoyd VC. Parents' participation in a work-based anti-poverty program can enhance their children's future orientation: Understanding pathways of influence. J Youth Adolesc 2013;42(6):777-91.

[72] Chaplin D, Capizzano J. Impacts of a summer learning program: A random assignment study of building educated leaders for life (BELL). Online Submission, 2006.

[73] Ferrari A, Aricò M, Dini G, Rondelli R, Porta F. Upper age limits for accessing pediatric oncology centers in Italy: A barrier preventing adolescents with cancer from entering national cooperative AIEOP trials. Pediatr Hematol Oncol 2012;29(1):55-61.

[74] Springer JF, Wright LS, McCall GJ. Family interventions and adolescent resiliency: The Southwest Texas State high-risk youth program. J Community Psychol 1997;25(5):435-52.

[75] Yu W. Educational experiment on primary school students' orientation and the longitudinal study. Tianjin Educ 10:13.

[76] Sigal AB, Wolchik SA, Tein JY, Sandler IN. Enhancing youth outcomes following parental divorce: A longitudinal study of the effects of the new beginnings program on educational and occupational goals. J Clin Child Adolesc Psychol 2012;41(2):150-65.

[77] Catalano RF, Fagan AA, Gavin LE, Greenberg MT, Irwin CE, Ross DA, et al. Worldwide application of prevention science in adolescent health. Lancet 2012;April:32-43.

[78] Shek DT, Ma CMS. Impact of the Project P.A.T.H.S. in the junior secondary school years: Objective outcome evaluation based on eight waves of longitudinal data. ScientificWorldJournal 2012. doi: 10.1100/2012/170345.

[79] Shek DT, Sun RCF. Development and evaluation of positive adolescent training through holistic social programs (PATHS) (Vol. 3). Singapore: Springer Science Business Media, 2013.

[80] Ullrich-French S, McDonough MH, Smith AL. Social connection and psychological outcomes in a physical activity-based youth development setting. Res Q Exerc Sport 2012;83(3):431-41.

[81] Ssewamala FM, Ismayilova L. Integrating children's savings accounts in the care and support of orphaned adolescents in rural Uganda. Soc Serv Rev 2009;83(3):453-72.

[82] Jorgensen SR. Project taking charge: An evaluation of an adolescent pregnancy prevention program. Fam Relat 1991;40(4):373-80.

[83] McNeal R, Handwerk ML, Field CE, Roberts MC, Soper S, Huefner JC, et al. Hope as an outcome variable among youths in a residential care setting. Am J Orthopsychiatry 2006;76(3):304-11.

[84] McCay BJ, Jones PJS. Marine protected areas and the governance of marine ecosystems and fisheries. Conserv Biol 2011;25(6):1130-3.

[85] Kirschman KJ, Roberts MC, Shadlow JO, Pelley TJ. An evaluation of hope following a summer camp for inner-city youth. Child Youth Care Forum 2010;39(6):385-96.

[86] Pittman K, Irby M. Preventing problems or promoting development: Competing priorities or inseparable goals. Takoma Park, MD: International Youth Foundation, 1996.

[87] Lai HH. China's western development program: Its rationale, implementation, and prospects. Mod China 2002;28(4):432-66.

[88] Shea M, Ma PW, Yeh CJ, Lee SJ, Pituc ST. Exploratory studies on the effects of a career exploration group for urban Chinese immigrant youth. J Career Assess 2009. doi: http://dx.doi.org/10.1177/1069072709334246.

[89] De Villiers M, Van den Berg H. The implementation and evaluation of a resiliency programme for children. S Afr J Psychol 2012;42(1):93-102.

[90] Huppert FA, Johnson DM. A controlled trial of mindfulness training in schools: The importance of practice for an impact on well-being. J Posit Psychol 2010;5(4):264-74.

[91] Storch EA, Arnold EB, Lewin AB, Nadeau JM, Jones AM, De Nadai AS, et al. The effect of cognitive-behavioral therapy versus treatment as usual for anxiety in children with autism spectrum disorders: A randomized, controlled trial. J Am Acad Child Adolesc Psychiatry 2013;52(2):132-42.

[92] Song Y. Study on the effect of coaching of secondary school students' academic aspirations on academic satisfaction. J Psychol Sci 2006;29(4):951-3.

[93] Yang X, Kong K. Study on the effect of the coaching of aspirations and attribution training on enhancing academic satisfaction. J Psychol Sci 2005;28(1):99-103.

[94] Wu FKY, Shek DT. A case study: Investigate the implementation of P.A.T.H.S. in a single school by analyzing the role of policy, program, people, process and place. Int J Adolesc Med Health 2012;24(3):201-6.

[95] Shea M, Ma WM, Yeh CJ. Development of a culturally specific career exploration group for urban Chinese immigrant youth. Career Dev Q 2007;56(1):62-73.

[96] Chung RCY. Hong Kong's smart identity card: Data privacy issues and implications for a post-September 11th America. Asia-Pacific Law Policy J 2003;4(2):519-68.

[97] Chung RCY, Bemak F. Group counseling with Asians. In: DeLucia-Waack J, Kalodner C, Riva M, eds. Handbook of group counseling and psychotherapy, 2nd ed. Thousand Oaks, CA: Sage, 2014:231-41.
[98] Hayman FM. Kids with confidence: A program for adolescents living in families affected by mental illness. Aust J Rural Health 2009;17(5):268-72.
[99] Shek DTL, Ma CMS. Impact of the Project P.A.T.H.S. in the junior secondary school years: Individual growth curve analyses. ScientificWorldJournal 2011;11:253-66.
[100] Metcalfe SA, Aitken M, Gaff CL. The importance of program evaluation: How can it be applied to diverse genetics education settings? J Genet Couns 2008;17(2):170-9.
[101] Leong FTL, Gim-Chung RH. Career assessment and intervention with Asian Americans. In: Leong FTL, ed. Career development and vocational behavior of racial and ethnic minorities. Hillsdale, NJ: Lawrence Erlbaum, 1995:193-226.

SECTION THREE: PSYCHOLOGICAL NEEDS AND RISK BEHAVIOR

In: Soft Skills and Aspirations … ISBN: 978-1-53614-092-7
Editors: Daniel TL Shek, et al.

Chapter 9

PSYCHOLOGICAL NEEDS, SELF-REGULATION, MOTIVATION AND HONG KONG CHINESE UNIVERSITY STUDENTS

Cecilia MS Ma[1,*], PhD,
Daniel TL Shek[1-5], PhD, FHKPS, BBS, JP and
Catie CW Lai[1], MAP, BSocSc

[1]Department of Applied Social Sciences,
The Hong Kong Polytechnic University, Hong Kong, PR China
[2]Centre for Innovative Programmes for Adolescents and Families,
The Hong Kong Polytechnic University, Hong Kong, PR China,
[3]Department of Social Work, East China Normal University,
Shanghai, PR China
[4]Kiang Wu Nursing College of Macau, Macau, PR China
[5]Division of Adolescent Medicine, Kentucky Children's Hospital,
University of Kentucky, Lexington, Kentucky, US

---

* Corresponding Author Email: cecilia.ma@polyu.edu.hk.

Abstract

To better understand factors that influence individuals' motivation to engage in physical activity, this study aimed to identify the motivational profiles among Chinese university students, compare the motivational profiles between genders and explore whether satisfaction of various psychological needs vary with different motivational profiles. A total of 2,022 Chinese university students completed a battery of self-report questionnaires assessing motivation regulation and psychological needs satisfaction. Three motivational profiles were identified for both genders, with the overall patterns of the motivational profiles for both genders similar. However, males (44%) were more likely than their female counterparts (19%) in self-determined profile group. Students with self-determined motivation profile, compared to non-self-determined motivation profile, had higher values on three types of needs satisfaction. Findings and implication of the study were discussed.

Introduction

Physical inactivity is one of the major health risk behaviors in college students (1) and has been identified as one of the priorities in the Healthy People 2010 objectives (2) and Healthy Campus 2010 Campaign Objectives (1). Health professionals and researchers call for the need to combat sedentary life among college students (3). Therefore, further research on this population is warranted to better understand factors that influence individuals' motivation to engage in physical activity.

Among numerous studies on sport and exercise motivation in literature, Self-determination theory (4, 5) is one of the widely used theoretical perspectives on the relationship between motivation and physical activity (6-8). According to SDT, motivations lie on a continuum from self-determined to non-self-determined, from intrinsic, external motivations to amotivation (9). Intrinsic motivation refers to individuals engage in physical activity because of inherent feelings, such as pleasure, fun and satisfaction, extrinsic motivation occurs when individuals decide to do exercise not because of inherent enjoyment (4). Extrinsic motivation is consisted of four types of regulation. They are integrated, identified, introjected and external, in descending order in the motivation continuum (4). Integrated regulation happens when participation in physical activity is to meet personal values, beliefs and goals. Identified regulation occurs when individuals participate in physical activity because they consider the activity valuable and important to themselves. Introjected regulation refers to participation in physical activity due to pressures, such as to avoid shame and guilt or to gain social recognition and feelings of worth. External regulation appears when participation in physical activity because of external demand or socially constructed contingency, such as reward, prize or punishment. At the self-determined bottom of the continuum is amotivation, which characterizes as a lack of intrinsic or extrinsic intention to do exercise (9). The fundamental premise of SDT is that self-determined motivation is facilitated by the social environment that provides satisfaction of three basic psychological needs, including relatedness (connectedness with others), competence (efficacy to complete an optimal challenge task) and autonomy (provision of choice, pressure-free, sense of volition) (9). Conversely, the social environment, thwarting these three needs, forestalls the internalization of behavioral regulation (9). Partial internalization occurs when the social environment provides satisfaction of competence and relatedness as the presence of autonomy is essential for full internalization (9). For example, they implied that the process of internalization can be forestalled, and therefore introjected regulation is fostered by satisfaction of needs for relatedness in an environment with external pressures and controls (i.e., absence of autonomy).

Koestner and Losier (10) supported that satisfaction of the need for autonomy is a chief element for progress in internalization. They, however, suggested different patterns of internalization by specifying the correlations between satisfaction of the three needs and introjected, identified and intrinsic behavioral regulations. Introjected and identified behavioral regulations are nurtured by satisfaction of the need for both autonomy and relatedness in a conflicting and harmonious environment, respectively. Instead of satisfaction of all three needs, relatedness is a less salient factor for promoting intrinsic regulation. Intrinsic regulation can occur in an environment providing support for competence and autonomy. Therefore, more research is warranted to examine the psychological needs for promoting self-determined motivation.

Research within the SDT framework has shown that a higher degree of self-determined behavioral regulation is related to the higher level of physical activity in cross-sectional (11, 12), longitudinal studies (13) and experimental studies (14). This is further supported by Teixeira and colleagues (15), who reviewed 66 empirical SDT studies, and found that self-determined motivation (i.e., intrinsic and identified regulation) is a significant predictor of more adaptive behavioral outcomes (exercise adherence, effort and persistence). However, prior studies were mainly conducted in western contexts without exploring gender difference on motivation.

First, there were very few studies examined the differences in motivation in non-western cultures. Duda and colleague (16,17) noted the role of culture in influencing individuals' cognition, affect and behavioral outcomes in physical activity research. SDT posits that culture is a critical factor influencing one's internalization that influences the development of autonomous regulations (self-determined motivation) and the decision making process (9). The emphasis on interdependence may influence the internalization of motivation in a collectivistic society (18). Individuals in eastern culture may be more internalized on conforming to the social norms and thus perceive such "action" as in line with their personal values. This may undermine the negative influence of the absence of autonomy, as posited in SDT (19). The presence of autonomy is less crucial on facilitating the process of internalization and promoting self-determined motivation in collectivistic and non-western contexts (20). Iyengar and Lepper (20) found that Asian individuals were more intrinsic motivated when the decision of participation in an activity was made by people they trusted, compared to personal choice. Given the cultural influence on internalization of motivation, it is vital to explore the relations between satisfaction of the three needs and the internalization of motivation.

Second, there are scarce studies adopting SDT framework to understand gender differences in motivation and needs satisfaction. Past studies showed that males were more likely to meet the American College of Sports Medicine guidelines of physical activity than females (21). This is further supported in Chinese samples (22, 23). Such gender differences may relate to the motivation to participate in physical activity. Research in education literature revealed that females displayed a more self-determined motivation and reported a lower level of dropout than their male counterparts (24). However, very few studies assess the gender differences in motivation regulations as a function of a greater amount of physical activity. To promote students' physical health, more research is warranted to examine factors (relatedness, competence and autonomy) that fostering internalization of behavioral regulation, so as to encourage more participation in and less dropout from physical activity.

Third, prior studies usually adopted a variable-centered approach in testing the relationships between each type of motivation and other variables. More specifically, a single indicator (i.e., Self-determination Index, SDI) is widely used to assess individual's motivation to participate in certain behavior (24-26). However, such method may fail to capture the multidimensionality of motivation and ignore the differences in the magnitude and direction of various patterns of correlations among motivation types. Moran and colleagues (27) argue that "this ignores the possibility that distinct constellations of motivational profiles exist in the population and these SDT motivation profiles may correspond to differences in other variables" (p. 354). A profile approach may provide unique information to study the relations between motivation and theoretically relevant antecedents and consequences. "Inconsistent support for the relationships of introjected and external regulations to theoretically relevant constructs may be due to examining regulation types in parallel rather than in combination" (28). Wang and colleagues suggest the use of person-oriented approach, such as latent profile analysis, to show how individuals differ in their motivational profile and the unique effect of each type of behavioral regulation on theoretically relevant factors (26, 29, 30). By using a person-centered approach, Moran, Diefendorff, Kim and Liu (27) found the self-determined and motivated groups perceived the greater satisfaction of the three needs, compared to the low introjection and low autonomy motivated groups. Therefore, more research is warranted to explore the diverse patterns of motivation in non-western contexts, possible differences in motivation profiles by gender and possible variations in satisfaction of the psychological needs among motivation profiles.

A person-oriented approach — Latent profile analysis (LPA)

Latent profile analysis (LPA), one of the person-centered approaches, assesses the latent structure of motivation and allows us to identify the homogeneous patterns of motivation groups of people who can be classified according to typologies. This method extends the traditional variable-centered research by considering intra-individual variation in motivation and capturing a better picture of an individual (31). LPA allows us to group individuals into profiles based on homogenous characteristics and to identify differences in satisfaction of psychological needs among different motivation profiles. Such research is beneficial for understanding how each motivation profile is uniquely related to other SDT variables.

In general, three motivational profiles (high self-determined, moderate self-determined and low self-determined/amotivated) were found in academic (32), physical education (33-35), and sports contexts (36). However, Cox and colleagues (34) recently found a four-cluster solution (highly diverse motivated, moderate motivated, moderate diverse motivated and externally motivated) when assessing the relationship between motivation profiles and outcomes affect (enjoyment), behavioral (effort) and cognitive (social physique anxiety) outcomes. Similarly, Moran and colleagues (27) explored the patterns of motivation and the linkages of each profile and outcomes (e.g., job performance, needs satisfaction) and found a five-cluster solution. Given the inconsistency of the motivational profiles in terms of quantity (number of profile/class membership) and quality (i.e., combination of different types of motivation regulation), further research in this area is warranted.

The purposes of the study were threefold: 1) to identify the motivational profiles among Chinese university students; 2) to compare the motivational profiles between male and female students; 3) to explore whether satisfaction of various psychological needs and vary with different motivational profiles. Based on the prior literature, high levels of self-determined motivation are expected to have higher perceptions of needs satisfaction.

OUR STUDY

A total of 2,022 Chinese participants (Male: n = 965, 47.7%; Female: n = 1,057, 52.2%) participated in the study. The participants were on average 18.73 (*SD* = 1.29). The majority of participants were Chinese (n = 1,896, 94%), freshmen (n = 1,952, 96.7%) and lived off-campus (n = 1,316, 65.5%).

Participants' level of motivation toward exercise was measured by the Behavioral Regulation in Exercise Questionnaire-2 (BREQ-2) (37). The scale comprises 19-items and measures an individual's 5 types of motivation, including intrinsic motivation (4 items), identified motivation (4 items), introjected regulation (3 items), external regulation (4 items) and amotivation (4 items). The study followed the practice as suggested by (32), integrated regulation whose identity is still undergoing formation, is not examined in our sample. Responses were indicated on a 5-point Likert-type scale ranging from 1 (*Strongly disagree*) to 5 (*Strongly agree*). Previous work has supported the construct validity and reliability of this scale (13). This scale has been used among college sample in Canada (39, 40) and the United Kingdom (40) and adults in Greece (41) and in the USA (42). The Cronbach's alphas of all subscales are satisfactory (identified regulation:

.75; external regulation: .80; introjected regulation: .75; intrinsic regulation: .86; amotivation: .86).

Psychological need satisfaction was assessed using the Psychological Needs Satisfaction in Exercise Scale (PNSES) (43). The scale comprises 18 items measuring three subscales including autonomy (6 items), competence (6 items) and relatedness (6 items). Responses are provided on a 6-point Likert scale, ranging from 1 (*Strongly disagree*) and 6 (*Strongly agree*). The validity and reliability of the scale has been shown in a prior study (44). This scale has been conducted among college sample in Canada (13, 38). The Cronbach's alphas of all subscales in the present study are satisfactory (competence: .94; autonomy: .89; relatedness: .91).

A back-translation procedure (45) was used to measure the meaning equivalence of the instrument. The original questionnaire was developed in English and translated into Chinese by the author who is fluent in both English and Chinese. Then, without referring to the original scale, backward translation was done by a professional Chinese translator, who is bilingually fluent in English and Chinese. Then, two independent researchers compared the backward translation version with the original version to ensure the content of both versions was the same. No deviation in meaning was found. The study received the approval of the University Human Research Ethics Committee. Informed consent was obtained before completing the questionnaire.

Descriptive statistics and internal consistency reliability were completed using SPSS version 22.0. All LPA models were performed using MPlus version 7.3. Multiple criteria were used to select the best-fitting model (46, 47), including the Akaike Information Criterion (AIC) the Bayesian Information Criterion (BIC) and the adjusted-BIC (ABIC). Lower values of these indices suggest better fit of the data. Also, the Lo-Mendell-Rubin test (LMRT) and Vuong-Lo-Mendell-Rubin (VLMRL) were employed to compare the increase in model fit between k-1 class and k class models. Significant p-values ($p < .05$) indicate a target model (k-class solution) fits the data better than the model with one fewer class (k-1 class solution) (48). Finally, entropy is inspected, ranging from 0 to 1 with higher values of entropy indicating better classification of individuals (49). Interpretability and theoretical appropriateness were also considered (31). Age was included as an auxiliary variable to investigate whether this demographic variable influences latent class assignment. This approach allowed us to decrease bias when estimating the parameters without influencing the model itself (50). In the present study, LPA was conducted separately for each gender group.

A latent profile solution

To perform latent profile analysis (LPA), all models were estimated in Mplus (version 7.30) by using maximum likelihood robust (MLR). Missing data was low (ranged from .3% to 1.6%, Table 1) and was estimated using an Expectation-Maximization (EM) Algorithm (50). Several solutions with 1-5 classes were tested to identify the optimal number of classes. Once the optimal number of motivational profiles is identified, a one-way multivariate analysis of covariance (ANCOVA) with Bonferroni adjustment post hoc test was used to test differences in needs satisfaction. Needs satisfaction served as dependent variables; motivational profile groups were the independent variable. Effect size of .01 is small, .06 is moderate, and .16 is high (51).

FINDINGS

All data were normally distributed (i.e., skewness < 2.0; kurtosis < 7.0) (52). Descriptive statistics and internal consistencies can be found in Table 1. To examine the factor structure of the BREQ-2 and PNSES, confirmatory factor analysis (CFA) was performed. A model is considered acceptable with a cut of criteria of a comparative fit index (CFI) of .90 or above (53, 54), a root mean square error of approximation (RMSEA) of .10 (55, 56) or below and a standardized root mean square residual (SRMR) with .08 or less (53). The factorial validity of the 3-factor correlated structure of the PNSES is supported, $\chi^2(132) = 2089.03$; $p < .01$, RMSEA=.09 (90% CI = .08-.09), CFI = .93, TLI = .92, SRMR = .05. The factor structure of the BREQ-2 showed a moderate fit of the 5-factor model, $\chi^2(142) = 2040.27$, RMSEA=.08 (90%

CI = .08-.08), CFI=.90, SRMR=.07. An inspection of the modification indices suggested the error variances of the two indicators of external regulation should be related (MI = 216.27). A modified model, therefore, was tested and showed a slightly improved fit, $\chi^2(141) = 1845.45$, RMSEA = .08 (90% CI = .07-.08, CFI = .91, SRMR = .07. The results of the CFA show the factorial validity of the BREQ-2. Internal consistency of all subscales is satisfactory (above .70, see Table 1).

Number of class

Male

Several models from 1-class to 5-class solutions were fitted (see Table 2). The 2-class solution was better than 1-class as indicated by lower BIC, AIC, ABIC and significant VLMR, LMRT. The 3-class solution was better than 2-class solution due to lower values of BIC, AIC and ABIC and a higher entropy value. Compared to the 5-class solution, the 4-class solution indicated better fit with higher Entropy. Despite the lower values of BIC, AIC and ABIC of the 4-class solution, the LMRT and VLRT were not statistically significant from the 3-class solution. Also, the 4-class and 5-class solutions were rejected as one of the profiles is less than 2% (i.e., 4-class: 1.2% of participants; 5-class: 1.5% of participants). Therefore, the 3-class solution was considered the best model. Entropy was .80 with average posterior probabilities ranged from .90-.93.

Female

Similar results were shown in the female group (see Table 3). The three-class solution fitted the data better as compared to the two-class solution due to the lower values of AIC, BIC and ABIC. The 4-class and 5-class solutions were rejected as one of the profiles with only 19 participants (less than 2%). A 3-class solution was, therefore, deemed optimal. Entropy .74 with class probabilities ranged from .87-.89.

Table 1. Descriptive statistics, internal consistencies and correlations of variables

	Whole	Male	Female	α	1	2	3	4	5	6	7	8
	M(*SD*)	*M*(*SD*)	*M*(*SD*)									
1. External	2.08 (.75)	2.02 (.74)	2.13 (.76)	.81	-							
2. Introjected	2.92 (.86)	2.98 (.88)	2.87 (.84)	.75	-.02	-						
3. Identified	3.53 (.78)	3.65 (.70)	3.41 (.68)	.75	-.18**	.68**	-					
4. Intrinsic	3.78 (.78)	4.02 (.71)	3.57 (.77)	.86	-.27**	.35**	.58**	-				
5. Amotivation	1.62 (.63)	1.58 (.63)	1.66 (.63)	.86	.57**	-.18**	-.39**	-.38**	-			
6. Competence	3.97 (1.09)	4.22 (1.04)	3.74 (1.07)	.94	-.21**	.31**	.50**	.61**	-.27**	-		
7. Autonomy	4.63 (.81)	4.75 (.78)	4.52 (.82)	.89	-.29**	.20**	.41**	.48**	-.37**	.53**	-	
8. Relatedness	4.18 (.94)	4.38 (.92)	3.99 (.92)	.91	-.16**	.36**	.53**	.69**	-.31**	.71**	.56**	-
Missing values (%)					.3	.4	.4	.3	.5	.4	.5	.6

$^{**}p < .01$.

Table 2. Results of latent profile analysis (LPA) for male

No. of class	AIC	BIC	ABIC	VLMR *p* value	LMR-A *p* value	BLRT *p* value	Entropy
1	10590.523	10638.832	10607.073	-	-	-	-
2	9902.420	9979.714	9928.899	.0000	.0000	<.0000	.695
3	9466.701	9572.980	9503.111	**.0461**	**.0489**	<.0000	.804
4	**9292.620**	**9427.885**	**9338.960**	.5466	.5526	<.0000	.854
5	**9012.086**	**9176.336**	**9068.356**	.0369	.0400	<.0000	.859

Note. AIC = Akaike Information Criterion; BIC = Bayesian Information Criterion; ABIC = Adjusted-BIC (ABIC); VLMR = Vuong-Lo-Mendell-Rubin-likelihood ratio test; LMR-A = Lo-Mendell-Rubin adjusted likelihood ratio test; BLRT = Bootstrapped likelihood ratio test.

Table 3. Results of latent profile analysis (LPA) for female

No. of class	AIC	BIC	ABIC	VLMR *p* value	LMR-A *p* value	BLRT *p* value	Entropy
1	11562.926	11612.222	11580.461	-	-	-	-
2	10767.986	10846.858	10796.040	< .0000	< .0000	< .0000	.695
3	10485.185	10593.635	10523.760	**.0216**	**.0233**	< .0000	.743
4	**10261.428**	**10399.455**	**10310.523**	.2270	.2339	< .0000	.798
5	**10052.685**	**10220.288**	**10112.301**	.3506	.3563	< .0000	.787

Note. AIC = Akaike Information Criterion; BIC = Bayesian Information Criterion; ABIC = Adjusted-BIC (ABIC); VLMR = Vuong-Lo-Mendell-Rubin-likelihood ratio test; LMR-A = Lo-Mendell-Rubin adjusted likelihood ratio test; BLRT = Bootstrapped likelihood ratio test.

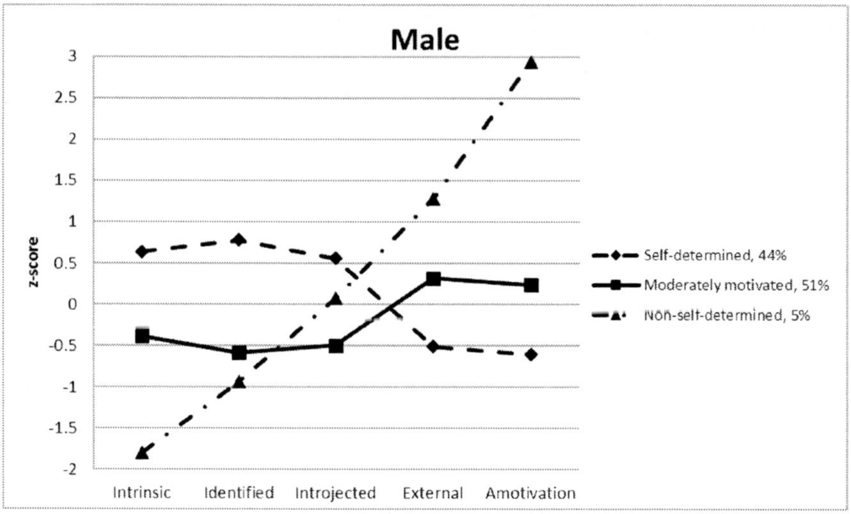

Figure 1. Profile characteristics with three latent classes for male.

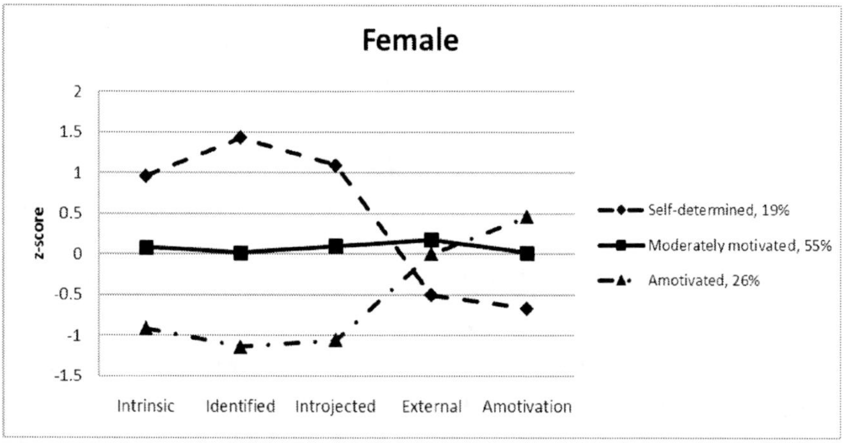

Figure. 2. Profile characteristics with three latent classes for female.

Motivational profiles

Male

The first class was named as moderately motivated group (n = 473, 51%). This class shows high intrinsic motivation (M = 3.73, SE = .05) and identified motivation (*M* = 3.27, *SE* = .04), moderate introjected motivation (*M* = 2.58, *SE* = .05) external regulation (*M* = 2.24, *SE* = .05) and external regulation (*M* = 2.24, *SE* = .05) and low amotivation (*M* = 1.77, *SE* = .06). The second class named as self-determined group (*n* = 408, 44%). This class shows high intrinsic motivation (*M* = 4.46, *SE* = .03), identified motivation (*M* = 4.20, *SE* = .05) and introjected (*M* = 3.48, *SE* = .08), low external regulation (*M* = 1.65, *SE* = .05) and amotivation (*M* = 1.20, *SE* = .03). The third class was named as non-self-determined group (*n* = 45, 5%). This class shows high amotivation (*M* = 3.72, *SE* = .30) and moderate external regulation (*M* = 2.96, *SE* = .15), low intrinsic motivation (*M* = 2.72, *SE* = .25), identified motivation (*M* = 3.02, *SE* = .17), and introjected motivation (*M* = 3.05, *SE* = .20). The inclusion of age as an auxiliary variable shows that age had no effect on the class assignment ($p > .05$).

Female

The first class was named as moderately motivated group (*n* = 558, 55%). This class shows moderate identified motivation (*M* = 3.43, *SE* = .09), intrinsic motivation (*M* = 3.63, *SE* = .07), introjected (*M* = 2.94, *SE* = .11) and external regulation (*M* = 2.27, *SE* = .05), low amotivation (*M* = 1.69, *SE* = .05). The second class was named as non-self-determined group (*n* = 263, 26%). This class shows moderate intrinsic motivation (*M* = 2.88, *SE* = .14), identified motivation (*M* = 2.68, *SE* = .08), external regulation (*M* = 2.16, *SE* = .06) and introjected (*M* = 2.03, *SE* = .09), low amotivation (*M* = 1.99, *SE* = .09). The third class was named as self-determined group (*n* = 201, 19%). This class shows high identified motivation (*M* = 4.35, *SE* = .10), intrinsic motivation (*M* = 4.31, *SE* = .06) and introjected (*M* = 3.78, *SE* = .10), low external regulation (*M* = 1.77, *SE* = .07) and amotivation (*M* = 1.25, *SE* = .05).

Age, as an auxiliary variable, had significant effect on the class assignment ($p < .05$). Results show that older females are likely to be classified in Classes 1 and 2 than in Class 3.

Class differences in need satisfaction

Three one-way multivariate analysis of covariance (MANCOVA) were performed to assess whether latent profile differed on motivation behavioral regulation and needs satisfaction.

Male

Age was entered as covariate, significant multivariate profile effect was found, $F(2, 894) = 75.37$, $p < .01$, Pillai's Trace, $\eta^2 = .43$ on external regulation, $F = 142.02, p < .01, \eta^2 = .24$), introjected ($F = 170.60$, $p < .01$, $\eta^2 = .28$), identified ($F = 455.49$, $p < .01$, $\eta^2 = .51$), intrinsic motivation ($F = 264.03$, $p < .01$, $\eta^2 = .37$), amotivation ($F = 470.26$, $p < .01$, $\eta^2 = .51$), competence ($F = 112.30$, $p < .01$, $\eta^2 = .20$), autonomy ($F = 96.86$, $p < .01$, $\eta^2 = .18$), relatedness ($F = 128.45$, $p < .01$, $\eta^2 = .22$). Age is not significant as covariate ($p > .05$). Post hoc tests showed that self-determined group reported higher levels of perceived competence than those in moderately self-determined motivated and amotivated groups ($p < .01$, Table 4). The differences between the moderately self-determined motivated and amotivated groups are not significant in perceived autonomy and perceived relatedness ($p > .01$).

Female

Significant profile effect was found ($F(2, 986) = 81.58$, $p < .01$, Pillai's Trace, $\eta^2 = .43$) on external regulation ($F = 37.44$, $p<.01$, $\eta^2 = .07$), introjected ($F = 556.33$, $p<.01$, $\eta^2 = .53$), identified ($F = 1182.08$, $p < .01$, $\eta^2 = .71$), intrinsic motivation ($F = 316.00$, $p < .01$, $\eta^2 = .39$), amotivation ($F = 88.38$, $p < .01$, $\eta^2 = .15$), competence ($F = 134.20$, $p < .01$, $\eta^2 = .21$), autonomy ($F = 88.98$, $p < .01$, $\eta^2 = .15$), relatedness ($F = 189.38$, $p < .01$, $\eta^2 = .28$). Age is not significant as covariate ($p > .05$). Post hoc tests showed that self-determined group reported highest levels of all outcome variables ($p < .01$, Table 4). The other two groups (i.e., amotivated and intrinsic and extrinsic motivated groups) did not differ in terms of all three types of needs satisfaction ($p > .01$). In general, regardless of gender, the magnitude of all profile differences was large (above .14) (52).

Table 4. Comparison of the three motivation profiles based on the motivation regulations for both genders

	Male								Female							
	Self-Determined (*n* = 408, 44%)		Moderately motivated (*n* = 473, 51%)		Non-self-determined (*n* = 45, 5%)				Self-determined (*n* = 201, 19%)		Moderately motivated (*n* = 558, 55%)		Non-self-determined (*n* = 263, 26%)			
	M(SE)	*Z*	*M(SE)*	*Z*	*M(SE)*	*Z*	*F*	η^2	*M(SE)*	*Z*	*M(SE)*	*Z*	*M(SE)*	*Z*	*F*	η^2
External	1.65 (.05)[ab]	-.51	**2.24 (.05)[a]**	**.32**	2.96 (.15)[b]	1.29	142.02**	.24	1.77 (.07)[a]	-.05	**2.27 (.05)[a]**	**.18**	2.16 (.06)[a]	.00	37.44**	.07
Introjected	**3.48 (.08)[a]**	**.56**	**2.58 (.05)[a]**	**-.49**	3.05 (.20)[a]	.08	170.60**	.28	**3.78 (.10)[a]**	**1.10**	**2.94 (.11)[a]**	**.10**	2.03 (.09)[a]	-1.05	556.33**	.53
Identified	**4.20 (.05)[a]**	**.78**	**3.27 (.04)[a]**	**-.58**	3.02 (.17)[a]	-.94	455.49**	.51	**4.35 (.10)[a]**	**1.43**	**3.43 (.09)[a]**	**.02**	**2.68 (.08)[a]**	**-1.14**	1182.08**	.71
Intrinsic	**4.46 (.03)[a]**	**.64**	**3.73 (.05)[a]**	**-.38**	2.72 (.25)[a]	-1.79	264.03**	.37	**4.31 (.06)[a]**	**.96**	**3.63 (.07)[a]**	**.08**	**2.88 (.14)[a]**	**-.91**	316.00**	.39
Amotivation	1.20 (.03)[a]	-.60	1.77 (.06)[a]	.24	**3.72 (.30)[a]**	**2.94**	470.26**	.51	1.25 (.05)[a]	-.66	1.69 (.05)[a]	.02	1.99 (.09)[a]	.46	88.38**	.15
Competence	4.74 (.05)[abc]	.48	3.83 (.04)[abc]	-.37	**3.25 (.19)[abc]**	**-.92**	112.30**	.20	4.50 (.07)[abc]	.07	3.78 (.04)[abc]	.05	3.03 (.06)[abc]	-.65	134.20**	.21
Autonomy	5.11 (.04)[abc]	.45	4.51 (.03)[abc]	-.33	**3.93 (.14)[abc]**	**-1.08**	96.86**	.18	5.09 (.05)[abc]	.71	4.48 (.03)[abc]	-.04	4.14 (.05)[abc]	-.46	88.98**	.15
Relatedness	4.85 (.04)[abc]	.50	4.05 (.04)[abc]	-.37	**3.33 (.16)[abc]**	**-1.16**	128.45**	.22	4.78 (.06)[abc]	.87	4.00 (.03)[abc]	.02	3.32 (.05)[abc]	-.71	189.38**	.28

Note. Entries with the same superscript indicate significant post-hoc differences in the Bonferroni test ($p < .01$).

Discussion

In this chapter we assess the motivational profile in both Chinese male and female university students. The three-cluster solution was aligned with prior findings in academic (32) and physical education contexts (33, 35). The overall patterns of the motivational profiles for both genders were similar. The majority of students belong to a moderately motivated profile. In this profile, students scored average in all forms of motivation regulations, except amotivation. In the second profile (self-determined profile), students scored high levels in self-determined motivation (i.e., intrinsic motivation and identified regulation), moderate levels of introjected regulation, and low levels of external regulation and amotivation. Students with self-determined motivation profile had higher values on three types of needs satisfaction. Consistent with the theoretical tenet of the SDT (9) and empirical findings, satisfaction of the three psychological needs motivation was a positive predictor to higher self-determined behavioral intention in physical activity (39). Furthermore, the current findings found males (44%) were more likely than their female counterparts (19%) in self-determined profile. This further supports the qualitative difference of motivational profiles of participants in physical activity contexts (28, 35).

Consistent with prior profile research (26, 35, 36), an amotivated group (non-self-motivated group) was found in both male and female groups. In this profile, students scored lowest in all needs (i.e., competence, autonomy, relatedness). Students from the amotivated group experienced lower satisfaction in all three needs of the SDT. This is worrisome, especially as 26% of females belong to this profile. This is consistent with a prior study, in which male Hong Kong Chinese college students reported higher level of physical activity than their female counterparts (22). These findings deserve our attention as previous research showed an inverse relationship between amotivation and effort in physical education (57), but no association with intention to exercise (58, 59).

The present study extends the literature about the importance of understanding qualitatively different reason to participate in a target behavior. “This way of identifying homogenous groups may be more realistic than artificially imposing a structure on the observed data" (36). Most previous work had not examined gender differences based on the mean score of each motivational regulation, except one academic study (24). Not much published physical activity research explored the motivational profiles in separate groups (gender: male and female). The present study extended prior studies by using a person-centered approach to explore the motivational regulation profiles among Chinese university students and to compare gender differences on the pattern of motivation profiles and its effects on SDT correlates (needs satisfaction).

Gender difference was found in the non-self-motived profile. The current study supported the proposition of the co-occurrence of two distinct motivations. By using this person-oriented approach, students reported optimal level of needs satisfaction when endorsing both high intrinsic (intrinsic and identified regulation) and moderate extrinsic motivations (introjected regulation). This was further supported by (60) who found that self-determined motivational profile (higher intrinsic motivation, identified regulation, introjected regulation and lower external regulation) was positively associated with perceptions of competence, autonomy and relatedness. This was consistent with academic research as conducted among high school (32) and college students (61). The present study extended SDT research, which was dominated by research using the variable-oriented approach and showed co-existence of both intrinsic and extrinsic motivations.

From a practical view, educators or practitioners should foster students' internalization and develop self-determined forms of behavioral regulations by establishing an autonomy-supportive learning atmosphere to motivate students to engage in physical activity, such as allowing them to participate in decision-making, providing an optimal achievable task, introducing peer learning group, building relationships with others and improving their understanding of the importance of physical activity, thereby promoting self-determined motivation towards physical activity. Researchers highlighted the role of culture in producing uniquely distinct SDT motivational profiles (27). More work should be replicated in different cultural contexts to assess the pattern of motivational profile and its impact on SDT correlates. For example, Moran and colleagues (27) identified a five-cluster solution of SDT profiles based on a sample of Chinese employees. However, it might be context-specific. Therefore, more research is warranted to increase the generalizability of the motivational research in physical activity contexts.

Several limitations were noted in the present study. First, the cross-sectional nature of the research design might limit the findings of the study. Future work might examine the temporal stability of these motivational profiles across time (62). Second, only antecedences were included. More studies are warranted to explore how the relationships between motivational regulations and its affective and behavioral outcomes would differ by gender. It is possible that behavioral outcomes, such as enjoyment, effort or level of physical activity, may differ among motivational profiles. Discriminant function analysis, (60) found that self-determined motivation predicted positive changes in exercise participation over time for both boys and girls. In particular, introjected regulation is a significant predictor to exercise behavior for boys, but not for girls. Lastly, more research is needed to see whether the present findings could be replicated in other non-western contexts, in which autonomy is less valued compared to western cultures (63).

Acknowledgments

This study was supported by the Start-up Fund for New Recruits from the Hong Kong Polytechnic University (account code: 1-ZE36). The materials in this paper are based on a paper published in the *International Journal on Disability and Human Development* 2017;16(4) issue.

References

[1] American College Health Association. Healthy campus 2010: make it happen 2002. URL: https://www.acha.org/healthycampus.

[2] Healthy people 2010: understanding and improving health. Washington, DC: US Dept. of Health and Human Services, 2000.

[3] Melton BF, Bigham LE, Bland HW, Bird M, Fairman C. Health-related behaviors and technology usage among college students. Am J Health Behav 2014;38(4): 510-8.

[4] Deci EL, Ryan RM. Intrinsic motivation and self-determination in human behavior. New York: Plenum, 1985.

[5] Deci EL, Ryan RM. The "what" and "why" of goal pursuits: human needs and the self-determination of behavior. Psychol Inq 2000;11(4):227-68.

[6] Edmunds J, Ntoumanis N, Duda JL. A test of self-determination theory in the exercise domain. J Appl Soc Psychol 2006;36(9):2240-65.

[7] Hagger M, Chatzisarantis N. Self-determination theory and the psychology of exercise. Int Rev Sport Exerc Psychol 2008;1(1):79-103.

[8] Mullan E, Markland D, Ingledew DK. A graded conceptualisation of self-determination in the regulation of exercise behaviour: development of a measure using confirmatory factor analytic procedures. Pers Individ Dif 1997;23(5):745-52.

[9] Deci EL, Ryan RM. Handbook of self-determination research. Rochester, NY: University of Rochester Press, 2002.

[10] Koestner R, Losier GF. Distinguishing three ways of being internally motivated: a closer look at introjection, identification, and intrinsic motivation. In: Deci EL, Ryan RM, editors. Handbook of self-determination research. Rochester, NY: University of Rochester Press; 2002:101-21.

[11] Owen KB, Astell-Burt T, Lonsdale C. The relationship between self-determined motivation and physical activity in adolescent boys. J Adolesc Health 2013;53(3):420-2.

[12] Sabiston CM, Brunet J, Kowalski KC, Wilson PM, Mack DE, Crocker PR. The role of body-related self-conscious emotions in motivating women's physical activity. J Sport Exerc Psychol 2010;32(4):417-37.

[13] Barbeau A, Sweet SN, Fortier M. A path-analytic model of self-determination theory in a physical activity context. J Appl Biobehav Res 2009;14(3):103-18.

[14] Standage M, Sebire SJ, Loney T. Engagement in objectively assessed bouts of moderate-intensity exercise: a self-determination theory perspective. J Sport Exerc Psychol 2008;30:337-52.

[15] Teixeira PJ, Carraça EV, Markland D, Silva MN, Ryan RM. Exercise, physical activity, and self-determination theory: A systematic review. Int J Behav Nutr Phys Act 2012;9(1):78-108.

[16] Duda JL, Allison MT. Cross-cultural analysis in exercise and sport psychology: a void in the field. J Sport Exerc Psycho 1990;12(2):114-31.

[17] Duda JL, Hayashi CT. Measurement issues in cross-cultural research within sport and exercise psychology. Adv Sport Exerc Psychol Meas 1998;7:471-83.

[18] Lonsdale C, Sabiston CM, Taylor IM, Ntoumanis N. Measuring student motivation for physical education: examining the psychometric properties of the perceived locus

of causality questionnaire and the situational motivation scale. Psychol Sport Exerc 2011;12(3):284-92.

[19] Deci EL, Koestner R, Ryan RM. A meta-analytic review of experiments examining the effects of extrinsic rewards on intrinsic motivation. Psychol Bull 1999;125(6):627-68.

[20] Iyengar SS, Lepper MR. Rethinking the value of choice: a cultural perspective on intrinsic motivation. J Pers Soc Psychol 1999;76(3):349-66.

[21] Martin SB, Morrow JR, Jackson AW, Dunn AL. Variables related to meeting the CDC/ACSM physical activity guidelines. Med Sci Sports Exerc 2000;32(12):2087-92.

[22] Lee RLT, Loke AJTY. Health-promoting behaviors and psychosocial well-being of university students in Hong Kong. Public Health Nurs 2005;22(3):209-20.

[23] Mok WK, Lee AYK. A case study on application of the theory of planned behaviour: predicting physical activity of adolescents in Hong Kong. J Community Med Health Educ 2013;3(5):231-7.

[24] Vallerand RJ, Fortier MS, Guay F. Self-determination and persistence in a real-life setting: toward a motivational model of high school dropout. J Pers Soc Psychol 1997;72(5):1161-76.

[25] Standage M, Duda JL, Ntoumanis N. Students' motivational processes and their relationship to teacher ratings in school physical education: a self-determination theory approach. Res Q Exerc Sport 2006;77(1):100-10.

[26] Wang CKJ, Biddle SJH. Young people's motivational profiles in physical activity: a cluster analysis. J Sport Exerc Psychol 2001;23:1-22.

[27] Moran CM, Diefendorff JM, Kim T-Y, Liu Z-Q. A profile approach to self-determination theory motivations at work. J Vocat Behav 2012;81(3):354-63.

[28] Ullrich-French S, Cox A. Using cluster analysis to examine the combinations of motivation regulations of physical education students. J Sport Exerc Psychol 2009;31(3):358-79.

[29] Lim BSC, Wang CKJ. Perceived autonomy support, behavioural regulations in physical education and physical activity intention. Psychol Sport Exerc 2009;10(1):52-60.

[30] Wang CKJ, Chatzisarantis NLD, Spray CM, Biddle SJH. Achievement goal profiles in school physical education: differences in self-determination, sport ability beliefs, and physical activity. Br J Educ Psychol 2002;72(3):433-45.

[31] Marsh HW, Lüdtke O, Trautwein U, Morin AJS. Classical latent profile analysis of academic self-concept dimensions: synergy of person- and variable-centered approaches to theoretical models of self-concept. Struct Equ Modeling 2009;16(2):191-225.

[32] Ratelle CF, Guay F, Vallerand RJ, Larose S, Senécal C. Autonomous, controlled, and amotivated types of academic motivation: a person-oriented analysis. J Educ Psychol 2007;99(4):734-46.

[33] Boiché J, Sarrazin PG, Grouzet FM, Pelletier LG, Chanal JP. Students' motivational profiles and achievement outcomes in physical education: a self-determination perspective. J Educ Psychol 2008;100(3):688.

[34] Cox AE, Ullrich-French S, Sabiston CM. Using motivation regulations in a person-centered approach to examine the link between social physique anxiety in physical education and physical activity-related outcomes in adolescents. Psychol Sport Exerc 2013;14(4):461-7.

[35] Ntoumanis N. Motivational clusters in a sample of british physical education classes. Psychol Sport Exerc 2002;3(3):177-94.

[36] McNeill MC, Wang CKJ. Psychological profiles of elite school sports players in Singapore. Psychol Sport Exerc 2005;6(1):117-28.

[37] Markland D, Tobin V. A modification to the behavioural regulation in exercise questionnaire to include an assessment of amotivation. J Sport Exerc Psycho 2004;26(2):191-6.

[38] Gunnell KE, Crocker PR, Mack DE, Wilson PM, Zumbo BD. Goal contents, motivation, psychological need satisfaction, well-being and physical activity: a test of self-determination theory over 6 months. Psychol Sport Exerc 2014;15(1):19-29.

[39] Wilson PM, Rodgers WM. The relationship between perceived autonomy support, exercise regulations and behavioral intentions in women. Psychol Sport Exerc 2004;5(3):229-42.

[40] Ingledew DK, Markland D, Ferguson E. Three levels of exercise motivation. Appl Psychol Health Well Being 2009;1(3):336-55.

[41] Vlachopoulos SP, Kaperoni M, Moustaka FC. The relationship of self-determination theory variables to exercise identity. Psychol Sport Exerc 2011;12(3):265-72.

[42] Markland D, Tobin VJ. Need support and behavioural regulations for exercise among exercise referral scheme clients: the mediating role of psychological need satisfaction. Psychol Sport Exerc 2010;11(2):91-9.

[43] Wilson PM, Rogers WT, Rodgers WM, Wild TC. The psychological need satisfaction in exercise scale. J Sport Exerc Psychol 2006;28(3):231-51.

[44] Gunnell KE, Wilson PM, Zumbo BD, Mack DE, Crocker PR. Assessing psychological need satisfaction in exercise contexts: Issues of score invariance, item modification, and context. Meas Phys Educ Exerc Sci 2012;16(3):219-36.

[45] Brislin RW. The wording and translation of research instruments. In: Lonner WJ, Berrhy JW, eds. Field methods in cross-cultural research. Beverly Hills, CA: Sage, 1986:137-64.

[46] Collins LM, Lanza ST. Latent class and latent transition analysis: with applications in the social behavioral, and health sciences. Hoboken, NJ: Wiley, 2010.

[47] Nylund KL, Asparouhov T, Muthén BO. Deciding on the number of classes in latent class analysis and growth mixture modeling: a monte carlo simulation study. Struct Equ Modeling 2007;14(4):535-69.

[48] Wang J, Wang X. Mixture modeling. In: Balding DJ, editor. Structural equation modeling: applications using mplus. New York: Wiley, 2012:289-390.

[49] Aldridge AA, Roesch SC. Developing coping typologies of minority adolescents: A latent profile analysis. J Adolescence 2008;31(4):499-517.

[50] Enders CK. A note on the use of missing auxiliary variables in full information maximum likelihood-based structural equation models. Struct Equ Modeling 2008;15(3):434-48.

[51] Cohen J. Statistical power analysis for the behavioral sciences, 2nd ed. Hillsdale, NJ: Lawrence Erlbaum, 1988.

[52] Curran PJ, West SG, Finch JF. The robustness of test statistics to nonnormality and specification error in confirmatory factor analysis. Psychol Methods 1996;1(1): 16-29.

[53] Hu LT, Bentler PM. Cutoff criteria for fit indexes in covariance structure analysis: conventional criteria versus new alternatives. Struct Equ Modeling 1999;6(1):1-55.

[54] Kline P. An easy guide to factor analysis. London: Routledge, 1994.

[55] Browne MW, Cudeck R. Alternative ways of assessing model fit. In: Bollen KA, Long JS, eds. Testing structural equation models. Newbury Park, CA: Sage, 1993:136-62.

[56] Byrne BM. Structural equation modeling with AMOS: basic concepts, applications, and programming. Mahwah, NJ: Lawrence Erlbaum, 2001.

[57] Shen B, Wingert RK, Li W, Sun H, Rukavina PB. An amotivation model in physical education. J Teach Phys Educ 2010;29(1):72-84.

[58] Standage M, Duda JL, Ntoumanis N. A model of contextual motivation in physical education: using constructs from self-determination and achievement goal theories to predict physical activity intentions. J Educ Psychol 2003;95(1):97-110.

[59] Taylor IM, Ntoumanis N, Standage M, Spray CM. Motivational predictors of physical education students' effort, exercise intentions, and leisure-time physical activity: a multilevel linear growth analysis. J Sport Exerc Psycho 2010;32(1):99-120.

[60] Gillison FB, Standage M, Skevington SM. Motivation and body-related factors as discriminators of change in adolescents' exercise behavior profiles. J Adolesc Health 2011;48(1):44-51.

[61] Smith JL, Deemer ED, Thoman DB, Zazworsky L. Motivation under the microscope: Understanding undergraduate science students' multiple motivations for research. Motiv Emot 2014;38(4):496-512.

[62] Hayenga AO, Corpus JH. Profiles of intrinsic and extrinsic motivations: A person-centered approach to motivation and achievement in middle school. Motiv Emot 2010;34(4):371-83.

[63] Markus HR, Kitayama S. Models of agency: Sociocultural diversity in the construction of action. In: Murphy-Berman V, Berman J, eds. Nebraska symposium on motivation: cross-cultural differences in perspectives on self. Lincoln, NE: University of Nebraska Press, 2003:1-57.

In: Soft Skills and Aspirations … ISBN: 978-1-53614-092-7
Editors: Daniel TL Shek, et al.

Chapter 10

EXPOSURE TO ONLINE PORNOGRAPHY AMONG HONG KONG CHINESE ADOLESCENTS

Cecilia MS Ma[1,*], PhD,
Daniel TL Shek[1-5], PhD, FHKPS, BBS, JP
and Catie CW Lai, MAP, BSocSc
[1]Department of Applied Social Sciences,
The Hong Kong Polytechnic University, Hong Kong, PRChina
[2]Centre for Innovative Programmes for Adolescents and Families,
The Hong Kong Polytechnic University, Hong Kong, PRChina
[3]Department of Social Work, East China Normal University,
Shanghai, PRChina
[4]Kiang Wu Nursing College of Macau, Macau, PRChina
[5]Division of Adolescent Medicine, Kentucky Children's Hospital,
University of Kentucky, Lexington, Kentucky, US

ABSTRACT

In this chapter, we tested how gender and religion affect exposure to unintentional and intentional exposure to online pornography in Chinese

---

* Corresponding Author Email: cecilia.ma@polyu.edu.hk.

adolescents. A total of 1,401 secondary school students (age range from 11 to 16 years) participated in the study. Findings based on multivariate analyses show that males reported higher levels of unintentional and intentional exposure to online pornography than females. Significant differences were found in adolescents' religiosity, with students having religious belief reported a lower level of unintentional exposure to online pornography than did their counterparts without religious belief. In terms of intentional exposure to online pornography, adolescents were more likely to be exposed if they were male and had religious beliefs. Such differences were not found in females. This study demonstrated the influence of demographic characteristics on exposure to online pornography among Chinese adolescents.

INTRODUCTION

The growing use of internet makes pornography more affordable and easier to access for adolescents (1-3). Nowadays, adolescents are frequent users of the internet for information, entertainment and communication (4-6). Indeed, the internet provides adolescents an ideal way to search for sexual information anonymously (3). This is particularly the case when they enter puberty and become more interested toward sex (7). Much of the previous research has focused on the negative impacts of pornography viewing, such as early sexual involvement (8), uncommitted sexual relationship (9), sexual victimization (8, 10), sexual permissiveness (11), objectification of women (12), substance abuse (13, 14), delinquency (10) low self-worth and depression (15). Research has been calling for identifying factors of pornography exposure in order to protect our adolescents against this behavior.

Gender is an important antecedent for exposure to online pornography (16). Males were generally found to be more frequent users of pornography (13, 17, 18), discuss more often about pornography with their peers (19), and perceive greater peer pressure to use pornography (20) than their female counterparts. Although literature generally supports that gender is an antecedent for exposure to online pornography, little is known about the consumption of different types of pornographic materials among males and females. Howard and colleagues found that males were more likely to participate in some online activities, such as joining a chat room and downloading a video or audio clip (21). Male internet users might be at higher risk of engaging in sexual chats or viewing pornographic videos. It is possible that males and females might search for different information or materials when using pornography. Therefore, systematic research on exposure to different types of pornographic materials by gender is needed.

Besides gender, religion is another possible factor influencing exposure to pornography. Many studies showed lower consumption of pornography was associated with adolescents who were studying in schools with religious background (15, 22-24) and attending religious services (15, 24). Moreover, prior research has demonstrated that religiosity was linked to self-regulation and self-control (22, 5), negative attitudes toward pornography (22, 26) and conformity to the social norms and expectations against watching pornography (22). These findings are also reported in a study examining religious communities (27). It seems that religion might promote more conservative attitude towards sex (26) and protect adolescents against pornography use (28). Nevertheless, prior studies addressing links between religion and pornography use are based on samples from Western contexts (22, 23). It is not clear whether this result can be generalized in non-western contexts. The aim of the present study was to explore how pornography use varies by religious backgrounds among Chinese adolescents.

Lastly, the nature of exposure has recently been studied in this area of research. Researchers suggested that as frequent users of the Internet, adolescents tend to be exposed to online pornography by chance (5, 18), such as some pop-up pornographic advertisements, when browsing the internet. Mitchell and colleagues (29) also noted that the wide availability of online pornography may lead to unintentional exposure to such materials. Recently, Peter and Valkenburg (30) conducted a systematic review of the literature on adolescents' consumption of pornography and highlighted the importance to distinguish between intentional and unintentional exposure of online pornography. It seems that factors linking to exposure to pornography may vary with viewers' intention when searching the internet. Therefore, studies for identifying factors related to exposure to online pornography should examine intentional and unintentional exposure separately.

In sum, the prevalence of the internet has led to an increase of exposure to online pornography. Adolescents are high-risk population to be exposed to online pornography due to increase curiosity towards sex and high frequency of internet use. Some demographic factors, such as gender and religiosity, have significant impacts on the frequency of exposure to online pornography. Recent literature suggests exposure to online pornography should be distinguished between intentional and unintentional exposure. Therefore, research on exposure to different types of pornographic materials by gender and with or without religious background is needed. There were two purposes of the present study. First, we explored the prevalence of intentional and unintentional online pornography among a sample of Chinese adolescents. Second, we examined whether the two types of exposure differed by gender and religious background.

OUR STUDY

A total of 1,401 Chinese secondary school students, including 753 males (54%) and 639 females (46%) were recruited from 13 secondary schools (age range from 11 to 16, M=12.43, SD=.70). Nine respondents failed to indicate their gender. Before data collection, students and their parents were contacted and informed about the purpose, procedures and confidentiality safeguards of the study. Ethical approval was obtained from the Hong Kong Polytechnic University Review Board. In general, it took around 15 minutes to complete the survey.

Six items were used to ask the frequency of unintentional exposure to six different types of online pornography materials, including (a) stories, b) pictures, c) videos, d) pornographic advertisement, e) websites, and f) chat room over the past half year. Same questions were asked about the frequency of intentional exposure to online pornographic materials. Responses ranged from (0 = never, 1 = less than once a month, 2 = once to three times a month, 3 = once a week, 4 = several times a week, and 5 = everyday). The internal consistency of both scales was satisfactory (unintentional: α=.78; intentional: α=.83).

Students answered three items to indicate their gender (0=male; 1=female), age and religiosity (0=yes; 1=no).

Independent *t*-tests were conducted to determine gender differences in mean score of twelve items of unintentional and intentional exposure to online pornography. Same analysis was performed to compare whether religiosity caused any differences in the items. To examine whether gender and religiosity jointly affected the two types of exposure to online pornography, a series of multivariate analysis of variance (MANCOVA) was tested by including an interaction term with two dichotomous variables (gender X religiosity) and age as covariate. All analyses were performed by SPSS for Windows (version 22.0).

OUR FINDINGS

The prevalence rates of the two types of exposure to online pornography are shown in Tables 1 and 2.

Table 1. Frequencies of intentional exposure to online pornography

Over the past six months, have you ever intentionally searched the internet to	Never	Less than once a month	1-3 times a month	About once a week	Several times a week	Daily
1) Read erotic stories (including comic stories)	90.1%	6.7%	1.8%	.7%	.4%	.4%
2) View pornographic pictures (showing genital areas/naked bodies)	85.9%	10.1%	2.1%	1%	.6%	.2%
3) View pornographic videos (including cartoon videos)	89.6%	7.2%	1.9%	.6%	.4%	.2%
4) Engage in sexual chats	95.8%	3%	.5%	.4%	.2%	.1%
5) View pornographic advertisement	87.2%	9.4%	2.1%	.7%	.4%	.2%
6) Browse pornographic websites	93.8%	4.4%	1%	.4%	.4%	.1%

About 4% (ranging from 2% to 6%) had unintentionally exposed themselves to online pornography, while 9% (ranging from 4% to 14%) of the respondents had intentionally exposed themselves to online pornography (see Table 1-2). In terms of intentional exposure, 14% (n=197) had viewed pornographic pictures and around 13% had watched pornography advertisement (n=179) in the past six months.

Table 2. Frequencies of unintentional exposure to online pornography

Over the past six months, while online, have you ever unintentionally been exposed to	Never	Less than once a month	1-3 times a month	About once a week	Several times a week	Daily
1) Erotic stories (including comic stories)	94.9%	2.9%	1.1%	.3%	.5%	.3%
2) Pornographic pictures (showing genital areas/ naked bodies)	94.7%	3.3%	1.1%	.4%	.4%	.1%
3) Pornographic videos (including cartoon videos)	93.6%	3.6%	1.7%	.5%	.5%	.1%
4) Sexual chatrooms	97.9%	1.4%	.1%	.1%	.3%	.1%
5) Pornographic advertisement	98.4%	1.4%	.1%	.1%	.1%	.1%
6) Pornographic websites	96.1%	2.3%	.9%	.3%	.4%	.1%

In Table 3, males reported higher levels of both types of exposure to online pornography (unintentional: 5-16%; intentional: 2-8%) than females (unintentional: 4-11%; intentional: 1-5%). In Table 4, students with religious beliefs reported lower levels of both types of exposure to online pornography (unintentional: 4-11%; intentional: 1-5%) than their counterparts with no religious beliefs (unintentional: 5-16%; intentional: 2-7%).

Table 3. Frequencies of unintentional and intentional exposure to online pornography by gender

	unintentionally		intentionally	
	Male	Female	Male	Female
1) Read erotic stories (including comic stories)	11.2%	8.3%	5.3%	4.7%
2) View pornographic pictures (showing genital areas/naked bodies)	16.4%	11.4%	6.4%	4.1%
3) View pornographic videos (including cartoon videos)	12.0%	8.5%	8.3%	4.4%
4) Engage in sexual chats	4.7%	3.8%	2.4%	2.7%
5) View pornographic advertisement	14.5%	11.0%	1.9%	1.4%
6) Browse pornographic websites	7.6%	4.5%	5.2%	2.5%

Table 4. Frequencies of intentional exposure to online pornography by religiosity

	unintentional		intentional	
	Yes	No	Yes	No
1) Read erotic stories (including comic stories)	6.8%	10.7%	4.2%	5.0%
2) View pornographic pictures (showing genital areas/ naked bodies)	11.0%	15.5%	4.0%	6.2%
3) View pornographic videos (including cartoon videos)	8.9%	11.2%	5.4%	6.7%
4) Engage in sexual chats	3.5%	5.0%	.7%	2.7%
5) View pornographic advertisement	10.1%	14.2%	.9%	2.3%
6) Browse pornographic websites	4.2%	7.6%	3.5%	4.6%

For unintentional exposure to online pornography, males reported significantly higher levels in all materials than females ($p < .05$), except visiting the chat room ($t_{(1387)} = 1.13, p > .05$, Table 5). Similarly, more males intentionally exposed themselves to pornographic pictures ($t_{(1388)} = 2.33, p < .05$, Table 5), videos ($t_{(1387)} = 3.03, p < .01$, Table 5) and website ($t_{(1387)} = 3.13, p < .01$). Adolescents' religiosity was significantly associated with their unintentional exposure to erotic stories ($t_{(1126)} = -2.27, p < .05$, Table 6), pornographic pictures ($t_{(1126)} = -2.42, p < .05$, Table 6). No significant difference was found in intentional exposure to online pornography, regardless of the sources ($p > .05$).

Table 5. Independent t-test results among the two types of exposure to pornographic materials by gender

	unintentional			intentional		
	Male	Female		Male	Female	
	M (SD)	*M* (SD)	*t*	*M* (SD)	*M* (SD)	*t*
1) Erotic stories (including comic stories)	.18 (.64)	.12 (.45)	2.19*	.11 (.54)	.08 (.40)	1.10
2) Pornographic pictures (showing genital areas/naked bodies)	.25 (.69)	.16 (.51)	2.64**	.11 (.51)	.06 (.32)	2.33*
3) Pornographic videos (including cartoon videos)	.18 (.60)	.12 (.48)	1.99*	.15 (.59)	.07 (.37)	3.02**
4) Sexual chatrooms	.08 .41)	.05 (.31)	1.13	.05 (.41)	.02 (.21)	1.59
5) Pornographic advertisement	.22 (.65)	.14 (.45)	2.52*	.03 (.25)	.01 (.12)	1.27
6) Pornographic websites	.12 (.50)	.06 (.32)	2.38*	.10 (.51)	.03 (.23)	3.13**

$^*p < .05$; $^{**}p < .01$.

Table 6. Independent t-test results among the two types of exposure to pornographic materials by religiosity

	unintentional			intentional		
	Yes	No		Yes	No	
	M (SD)	*M* (SD)	*t*	*M* (SD)	*M* (SD)	*t*
Erotic stories (including comic stories)	.10 (.42)	.17 (.59)	-2.27*	.08 (.42)	.09 (.50)	-.61
Pornographic pictures (showing genital areas/naked bodies)	.15 (.51)	.24 (.70)	-2.42*	.09 (.48)	.10 (.45)	-.44
Pornographic videos (including cartoon videos)	.14 (.52)	.18 (.60)	-1.13	.10 (.50)	.12 (.52)	-.51
Sexual chatrooms	.05 (.30)	.08 (.39)	-1.22	.02 (.28)	.04 (.32)	-1.17
Pornographic advertisement	.15 (.55)	.21 (.60)	-1.58	.01 (.17)	.03 (.25)	-1.19
Pornographic websites	.07 (.40)	.12 (.48)	-1.62	.08 (.48)	.07 (.40)	.33

*$p < .05$.

Table 7. Differences in unintentional exposure to online pornography by gender

Gender			
Male	Female	F	η2
M (SD)	*M* (SD)	5.55*	.005
.17 (.43)	.11 (.30)		

*p < .05.

Table 8. Differences in unintentional exposure to online pornography by religiosity

Religious			
Yes	No	F	η2
M (SD)	*M* (SD)	6.49*	.000
.11 (.29)	.16 (.42)		

*$p < .05$.

The interaction effect of gender and religion was not significant in unintentional exposure to online pornography ($F_{(1, 1111)}$ =.05, $p > .05$). Significant differences were found in gender ($F_{(1, 1112)}$ =5.55, $p < .05$, η^2=.005, Table 7) and religiosity ($F_{(1, 1112)}$ =6.49, $p < .05$, η^2=.006, Table 8). As expected, a majority of males reported higher level of unintentionally exposure to online pornography (*M* = .16, *SE* = .02) than females did (*M* = .11, *SE* = .02). Also, students with religious background had a lower level of such exposure (*M* = .10, *SE* = .02) than those without religious background (*M* = .16, *SE* = .02).

Based on the MANCOVA results, a significant interaction effect of gender and religious beliefs was found in intentional exposure ($F_{(1, 1111)}$ =4.32, $p < .05$, η^2=.004, Table 9). For intentional exposure, females with religious belief reported a lower level of mean score (*M* = .01, *SE* = .02) than their non-religious counterparts (*M* = .07, *SE* = .02). Conversely, males with religious belief showed a higher level of intentionally exposure to online pornography (*M* = .11, *SE* = .02) than their counterparts with no religious belief (*M* = .08, *SE* = .02). These results are shown in Figures 1 and 2. Linear regression models were performed to test the predictive effects of gender and religion on both types of exposure to online pornography. In Table 10, results showed that gender was significantly associated with both unintentional (β = -.08, $p < .01$) and intentional exposure (β = -.07, $p < .05$) to online pornography. Regardless of the nature of exposure, females were less likely to be exposed to this material than males. Religion had significant predictive effect on unintentional exposure (β = -.07, $p < .05$) but not in intentional exposure (β = -.02, $p > .05$) to online pornography. Adolescents, particularly those with religious beliefs, were more likely to be unintentionally exposed to pornographic material than those without religious beliefs.

Table 9. MACOVA results of the two types of exposure to online pornography by religiosity and gender

	Yes		No		F	ŋ2
	Male	Female	Male	Female		
	M (SD)	*M* (SD)	*M* (SD)	*M* (SD)		
Unintentional	.13 (.34)	.19 (.47)	.08 (.22)	.13 (.35)	.05	.000
Intentional	.11 (.40)	.08 (.36)	.01 (.08)	.07 (.26)	4.32*	.004

*$p < .05$;

Table 10. Linear regression models predicting unintentional and intentional exposure to online pornography by religiosity

	unintentional			intentional		
Predictor	R	R^2	β^a	R	R^2	β^a
Gender			-.08**			-.07*
Religiosity			-.07*			-.02
Model	.11	.01		.07	.01	

[a] Standardized coefficients.
$p < .05^*$, $p < .01^{**}$.

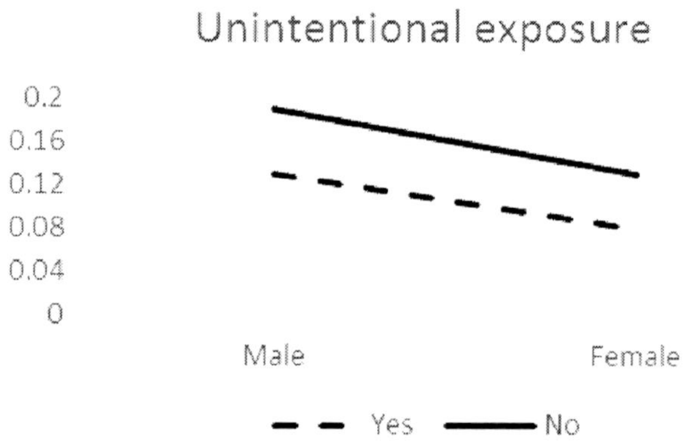

Figure 1. Unintentional exposure to online pornography by gender and religiosity.

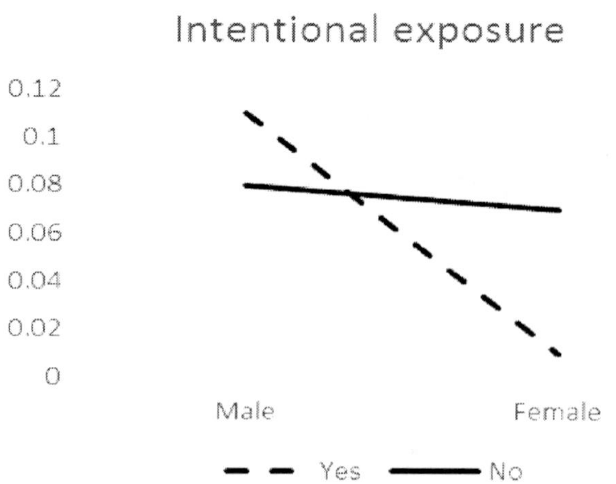

Figure 2. Intentional exposure to online pornography by gender and religiosity.

Discussion

The current study extends the scientific literature on consumption of pornographic materials in three ways. First, contrary to prior studies (10), adolescents reported more unintentional exposure to pornography than intentional exposure. However, it is important to note that the prevalence rates for intentional and unintentional exposure are generally low (unintentional: 4-14%; intentional: 2-6%), compared to studies conducted in Australia (84% males, 60% females (aged 16-17 years) were unintentionally exposed) (8), Taiwan (41% unintentional and 59% intentional among Grade 10-12 students) (31), and the United States (63% intentional and 32% unintentional among 15-18 adolescents) (22).

One possible reason might be related to the age of our sample. Sex is considered as taboo in Chinese society. Viewing pornography, even unintentionally, is undesirable and contradicts with traditional Chinese values (32). Given that the majority of the participants of the present study were early adolescents, they might be embarrassed to admit they were intentionally exposed to pornographic material. More research in exploring the prevalence of both types of online pornography use is suggested.

Second, adolescents with religious beliefs reported a lower level of unintentional exposure to online pornography than their counterpart without religious beliefs. Uecker (27) suggested that religion might serve as another way of social control against negative behaviors. Prior studies showed that religious youth has a higher level of self-regulation (33), greater self-control (25), a lower level of risky sexual behavior (34, 35), and they are less likely to use pornography (intentionally or unintentionally) (15, 22, 23). Religious beliefs also help adolescents to form "correct" sexual values such as respecting the body of the opposite sex and "inappropriateness" of seeing the bodies of the opposite sex outside marriage. The present findings extend the literature by demonstrating the protective effects of religion against negative behavior in a non-western culture.

Third, interestingly, the link between intentional exposure to online pornography and religiosity varied with gender. Aligned with previous literature, the protective effect of religiosity was found in females. In contrast, compared to males without a religious background, males with religious beliefs showed a greater level of being intentionally exposed to online pornography. Religiosity has long been posited as a factor contributing to more conservative attitude toward sexuality (26). Although males with religious beliefs are being stimulated by their sexual interest and curiosity, they face social pressure to abstain from their sexual needs. Instead of exploring their sexual identity in real life, they actively search for online pornography, which provides them "a protective cloak of anonymity" to disclose themselves (36) and to obtain emotional support from others (37). The present study highlights the interaction of demographic characteristics when studying the antecedents of this behavior. Future research should explore the effects of different combinations of demographic factors on the use of online pornography.

Several limitations should be noted for this study. First, as our findings were based on a cross-sectional design, causal relationships between the antecedents and exposure to online pornography cannot be concluded. Future study using a longitudinal design would help uncover the correlates and its influences on both types of exposure to online pornography. Second, the nature of internet activity might affect the frequency of intentional and unintentional exposure to online pornography. Ševčíková and colleagues (38) found that gender was significantly related to unintentional exposure to online pornography when adolescents visited X-rated and peer-to-peer sharing websites, but not in social networking sites. Perhaps, the nature of online activities should be included when studying how gender is related to exposure to online pornography. The present study did not examine their involvement and internalization of religiousness. A prior study found that these factors exerted protective effects on adolescents' consumption of pornography (22). More work is warranted to investigate the influence of different aspects of religiousness on pornography viewing.

In conclusion, the current study showed lower levels of unintentional and intentional exposure to online pornography at a younger age among Chinese adolescents. Regarding the frequency of exposure, male adolescents with a religious background were likely to be more frequently exposed to online pornography. Perhaps, the secrecy and solitary nature of the internet provided an ideal place to satisfy this target population's needs and curiosity due to their higher interest in sexuality. Further, this study provides support for arguments on the necessity to differentiate the nature of exposure to online pornography (22, 23). Lastly, the present findings identified the protective role of religion and suggested the possibility for using religion when designing sexual prevention program for Chinese adolescents.

ACKNOWLEDGMENTS

The present study is funded by a grant (Grant no. 25401414) of the Early Career Scheme of the Research Grants Council of the University Grants Committee of Hong Kong. The materials in this paper are based on a paper published in the *International Journal on Disability and Human Development* 2017;16(4) issue.

REFERENCES

[1] Beaver W. The dilemma of internet pornography. Bus Soc Rev 2000;105(3):373-82.

[2] Buzzell T. The effects of sophistication, access and monitoring on use of pornography in three technological contexts. Deviant Behav 2005;26(2):109-32.

[3] Cooper A. Sexuality and the internet: surfing into the new millennium. Cyberpsychol Behav 1998;1(2):187-93.

[4] Lenhart A, Maddenn M, Hitlin P. Teens and technology: youth are leading the transition to a fully wired and mobile nation. Washington, DC: Pew Internet American Life Project, 2005.

[5] Livingstone S, Helsper EJ. Taking risks when communicating on the internet: the role of offline social-psychological factors in young people's vulnerability to online risks. Inform Commun Soc 2007;10(5):619-44.

[6] Mesch G, Talmud I. The quality of online and offline relationships: the role of multiplexity and duration of social relationships. Inform Soc 2006;22(3):137-48.

[7] Flannery DJ, Rowe DC, Gulley BL. Impact of pubertal status, timing, and age on adolescent sexual experience and delinquency. J Adolesc Res 1993;8(1):21-40.

[8] Flood M. Exposure to pornography among youth in Australia. J Sociol 2007;43(1): 45-60.

[9] Byrne D, Osland JA. Sexual fantasy and erotica/pornography: internal and external imagery. Psychol Pers Hum Sex 2000:283-305.

[10] Wolak J, Mitchell K, Finkelhor D. Unwanted and wanted exposure to online pornography in a national sample of youth Internet users. Pediatrics 2007;119(2): 247-57.

[11] Braun-Courville DK, Rojas M. Exposure to sexually explicit web sites and adolescent sexual attitudes and behaviors. J Adolesc Health 2009;45(2):156-62.

[12] Peter J, Valkenburg PM. Adolescents' exposure to a sexualized media environment and their notions of women as sex objects. Sex Roles 2007;56(5-6):381-95.

[13] Carroll JS, Padilla-Walker LM, Nelson LJ, Olson CD, Barry CM, Madsen SD. Generation XXX pornography acceptance and use among emerging adults. J Adolesc Res 2008;23(1):6-30.

[14] Svedin CG, Åkerman I, Priebe G. Frequent users of pornography: a population based epidemiological study of Swedish male adolescents. J Adolesc 2011;34(4):779-88.

[15] Nelson LJ, Padilla-Walker LM, Carroll JS. "I believe it is wrong but I still do it": a comparison of religious young men who do versus do not use pornography. Psychol Relig Spiritual 2010;2(3):136-47.

[16] Vandenbosch L. Antecedents of adolescents' exposure to different types of sexually explicit Internet material: a longitudinal study. Comput Human Behav 2015;50: 439-48.

[17] Traeen B, Spitznogle K, Beverfjord A. Attitudes and use of pornography in the Norwegian population 2002. J Sex Res 2004;41(2):193-200.

[18] Ybarra ML, Mitchell KJ. Exposure to internet pornography among children and adolescents: a national survey. Cyberpsychol Behav 2005;8(5):473-86.

[19] Vanden Abeele M, Campbell SW, Eggermont S, Roe K. Sexting, mobile porn use, and peer group dynamics: boys' and girls' self-perceived popularity, need for popularity, and perceived peer pressure. Media Psychol 2014;17(1):6-33.

[20] Weber M, Quiring O, Daschmann G. Peers, parents and pornography: exploring adolescents' exposure to sexually explicit material and its developmental correlates. Sex Cult 2012;16(4):408-27.

[21] Howard PE, Rainie L, Jones S. Days and nights on the internet. In: Wellman B, Haythornwaite C, eds. The internet in everyday life. Oxford, UK: Blackwell, 2002: 45-74.

[22] Hardy SA, Steelman MA, Coyne SM, Ridge RD. Adolescent religiousness as a protective factor against pornography use. J Appl Dev Psychol 2013;34(3):131-9.

[23] Mesch GS. Social bonds and internet pornographic exposure among adolescents. J Adolesc 2009;32(3):601-18.

[24] Stack S, Wasserman I, Kern R. Adult social bonds and use of Internet pornography. Soc Sci Q 2004;85(1):75-88.

[25] McCullough ME, Willoughby BLB. Religion, self-regulation, and self-control: associations, explanations, and implications. Psychol Bull 2009;135(1):69-93.

[26] Regnerus MD. Forbidden fruit: Sex and religion in the lives of American teenagers. Oxford: Oxford University Press, 2009.

[27] Uecker JE. Religion, pledging, and the premarital sexual behavior of married young adults. J Marriage Fam 2008;70(3):728-44.

[28] Sherkat DE, Ellison CG. The cognitive structure of a moral crusade: conservative Protestantism and opposition to pornography. Soc Forces 1997;75(3):957-80.

[29] Mitchell KJ, Finkelhor D, Wolak J. The exposure of youth to unwanted sexual material on the internet a national survey of risk, impact, and prevention. Youth Soc 2003;34(3):330-58.

[30] Peter J, Valkenburg PM. Adolescents and pornography: a review of 20 years of research. J Sex Res 2016;53(4-5):509-31.

[31] Chen AS, Leung M, Chen CH, Yang SC. Exposure to internet pornography among taiwanese adolescents. Soc Behav Pers 2013;41(1):157-64.

[32] Thornburgh D, Lin HS. Youth, pornography, and the internet. Washington, DC: National Academies Press, 2002.

[33] Crockett LJ, Raffaelli M, Shen YL. Linking self-regulation and risk proneness to risky sexual behavior: pathways through peer pressure and early substance use. J Adolesc Res 2006;16(4):503-25.

[34] Dowshen N, Forke CM, Johnson AK, Kuhns LM, Rubin D, Garofalo R. Religiosity as a protective factor against HIV risk among young transgender women. J Adolesc Health 2011;48(4):410-4.

[35] Ogland CP, Xu X, Bartkowski JP, Ogland EG. The association of religion and virginity status among Brazilian adolescents. J Adolesc Health 2011;48(6):651-3.

[36] McKenna KY, Bargh JA. Plan 9 from cyberspace: The implications of the Internet for personality and social psychology. Pers Soc Psychol Rev 2000;4(1):57-75.

[37] Derlega VJ, Metts S, Petronio S, Margulis ST. Self-disclosure. Thousand Oaks, CA: Sage, 1993.

[38] Ševčíková A, Daneback K. Online pornography use in adolescence: age and gender differences. Eur J Dev Psychol 2014;11(6):674-86.

In: Soft Skills and Aspirations … ISBN: 978-1-53614-092-7
Editors: Daniel TL Shek, et al.

Chapter 11

PROTECTIVE FACTORS OF INTENTIONAL AND UNINTENTIONAL CONSUMPTION OF ONLINE PORNOGRAPHY IN HONG KONG

Cecilia MS Ma[1,*], PhD,
Daniel TL Shek[1-5], PhD, FHKPS, BBS, JP
and Catie CW Lai, MAP, BSocSc
[1]Department of Applied Social Sciences,
The Hong Kong Polytechnic University, Hong Kong, PR China
[2]Centre for Innovative Programmes for Adolescents and Families,
The Hong Kong Polytechnic University, Hong Kong, PR China
[3]Department of Social Work, East China Normal University,
Shanghai, PR China
[4]Kiang Wu Nursing College of Macau, Macau, PR China
[5]Division of Adolescent Medicine, Kentucky Children's Hospital,
University of Kentucky, Lexington, Kentucky, US

[*] Corresponding Author Email: cecilia.ma@polyu.edu.hk.

Abstract

In this chapter, we explore how positive youth development and family functioning were related to unintentional and intentional exposure to online pornography in Chinese adolescents. A total of 1,401 secondary school students (mean age = 12.43) participated in the study. Findings suggested that higher positive youth development and family functioning were associated with lower exposure to online pornography. In particular, higher levels of spirituality, social competence, mutuality, and communication were associated with lower levels of both types of exposure to online pornography. Discussion focuses on the importance of promoting positive youth development and family functioning as protective factors against the negative influence of pornography among Chinese adolescents.

Introduction

With the advent of the internet, the influence of pornography became a significant concern for parents, teachers and policymakers because adolescents often consume pornographic materials when surfing the internet. Prevalence of online pornography consumption varies greatly, ranging from 16% among Chinese adolescents (1) to almost 80% in German adolescents (93% of boys and 61% girls) (2). Such variation might be due to the failure to distinguish between intentional and unintentional exposure to pornography.

Indeed, the nature of exposure has recently become a central focus in this area of research. For example, about 70% of adolescents had been unintentionally exposed to online pornography in the United States (3) and Australia (4), while around four tenths of the adolescents had such experiences in Taiwan (5). Mesch argued that "as the negative consequences of exposure to pornography depend on the frequency of use, characteristics of adolescents at risk of deliberate exposure to pornography need to be identified, and distinguished from those of other youth who use the Internet for more socially acceptable purposes" (6). Unfortunately, although research of the influence of pornography is attracting increasing attention, we know very little about the correlates of these two types of exposure to online pornography. There are different theoretical views on the role of pornography consumption in adolescence. For those adhering to Freudian ideas, they tend to maintain that consumption helps to release tension. However, consuming pornography is also considered a risk factor as adolescents usually engage in other problematic behaviors simultaneously, such as substance abuse (7, 8) and breaking rules (3). With reference to the latter view, there is a need to understand factors linking to intentional and unintentional exposure to online pornography.

Numerous studies indicated the negative outcomes of pornography viewing, such as increased permissive attitudes toward sex (9, 10), acceptance of sexual aggression (11) and sexual dissatisfaction (12, 13). However, few research studies have been conducted to examine the protective factors to adolescent pornography use. There has been a growing literature assessing the protective factors, with a recent focus on how individual and family factors may influence exposure to online pornography. Much of the literature has been found that positive youth development is related to lower odds of adolescent gambling (14), sexual activity/intention, drug abuse (15), intention to engage in risky behavior (16) and delinquency (17). It is posited that developing adolescent competence and strengths would help them minimize the occurrence of behavioral problems and serve to mediate the relationship between life satisfaction and problem outcomes (18). The positive impacts of positive youth development were well-documented in cross-sectional and longitudinal studies. However, not much has been done to assess whether the protective function of this factor varies across two types of exposure to online pornography. The present study attempted to fill this research gap.

Another potentially important protective factor against pornography viewing is family functioning. There is a substantial body of research showing family functioning is a protective factor for adolescents. Higher family functioning is associated with better psychological well-being (19) and lower likelihood of problematic behaviors, such as substance abuse (20), suicide attempt (21), delinquent behavior (22, 23), and gambling (24). Recent findings have shown that family functioning reduced the likelihood of pornography viewing among adolescents (25, 26). This link has been later supported in longitudinal studies when testing the relationship between family functioning at Grade 7 and pornography use at Grade 9 (27) and at

Grade 10 (1). However, little is known whether these associations vary with the nature of exposure. Hence, a better understanding of the conditions of pornography viewing should provide the means for identifying protective factors to help educators and practitioners to design policies and programs for protecting adolescents against the negative influence of pornography.

There were two purposes of the present study. First, we explored how positive youth development and family functioning affected adolescents' exposure to online pornography. Second, we compared whether there was any difference between the unintentional and intentional nature of the exposure.

OUR STUDY

Completed questionnaires were collected from 1,401 Hong Kong Chinese secondary school students (753 males and 639 females, mean age = 12.43). Nine respondents did not indicate their gender. Participants were recruited from 13 schools, located in Hong Kong Island, Kowloon and New Territories. The questionnaire was administered by a trained research assistant and took around 15 minutes to complete. Ethical approval for the study was obtained from the Hong Kong Polytechnic University institutional review board.

Positive youth development was assessed with students' reports on the short form of the Chinese Positive Youth Development Scale (CPYDS). Item-scale ranged from (1 = strongly disagree to 6 = strongly agree). Based on prior measurement invariance results (28), the 15 subscales of the CPYDS were explained by four second-order factors, including cognitive-behavioral competencies, prosocial attributes, positive identity and general positive youth development qualities. In the present study, only the general positive youth development qualities with eight first-order factors (bonding resilience, social competence, recognition for positive behavior, emotional competence, moral competence, self-efficacy, and spirituality) were used. The scale showed good internal consistency. In Table 1, the internal consistency of this scale was satisfactory (total scale: α = .82, ranging from .71-.84 for subscales), except for self-efficacy (α = .61).

Table 1. Descriptive statistics, internal consistency and correlations among variables

	Mean	SD	α	1	2	3	4	5	6	7	8	9	10	11	12	13	14	15
BO	4.63	.86	.73	-														
RE	4.60	.91	.79	.50**	-													
SC	4.75	.88	.84	.48**	.53**	-												
PB	4.41	.92	.73	.64**	.44**	.50**	-											
EC	4.33	.96	.76	.46**	.55**	.56**	.46**	-										
MC	4.34	.90	.72	.47**	.53**	.50**	.45**	.63**	-									
SE	4.26	.96	.61	.43**	.48**	.44**	.42**	.46**	.56**	-								
SP	5.01	1.24	.74	.48**	.52**	.35**	.39**	.39**	.36**	.39**	-							
Mutuality	3.86	.91	.87	.49**	.35**	.34**	.34**	.39**	.36**	.33**	.49**	-						
Harmony	3.78	.91	.71	.31**	.23**	.20**	.23**	.22**	.20**	.18**	.31**	.59**	-					
Com	3.52	.99	.80	.49**	.37**	.32**	.36**	.37**	.37**	.33**	.48**	.76**	.45**	-				
PYD	4.57	.71	.82	.75**	.78**	.73**	.73**	.77**	.76**	.69**	.70**	.54**	.33**	.54**	-			
CFAI	3.72	.81	.89	.50**	.37**	.34**	.36**	.38**	.36**	.33**	.50**	.92**	.79**	.87**	.55**	-		
INV	.14	.36	.78	-.10**	-.11**	-.10**	-.10**	-.11**	-.13**	-.05	-.10**	-.13**	-.08**	-.10**	-.15**	-.12**	-	
VN	.07	.27	.83	-.07*	-.05	-.06*	-.06*	-.08**	-.11**	-.03	-.06*	-.09**	-.06*	-.03	-.11**	-.07**	.54**	-

Note: BO: bonding; RE: resilience; SC: social competence; PB: recognition for positive behavior; EC: emotional competence; MC: moral competence; SD: self-determination; SE: self-efficacy; SP: spirituality; Com: Communication; PYD: total score of the positive youth development qualities; CFAI: total score of family functioning; INV: unintentional exposure to pornography; VN: intentional exposure to pornography; $p < .05$*, $p < .01$**.

Students' perception on their family functioning was assessed using the modified version of Chinese Family Assessment Instrument (CFAI). Students were asked about the three aspects of family functioning, including mutuality (mutual support, love, and concern among family members), communication (frequency and nature of interaction among family members), conflicts and harmony (absence of conflicts and harmonious behavior in the family) were examined. This nine-item scale shows good internal consistency and validity (29). In the present study, the internal consistency of the scale was satisfactory ($\alpha = .89$; ranging from .71 to .87 for subscales, see Table 1). Participants were asked to answer their age, gender and place of birth. Item inter-correlations and Cronbach α coefficients were calculated as a measure of reliability. Associations were examined using Pearson r correlations. Linear regression models were conducted for exploration of the effects of variables. The data were analyzed by using IBM SPSS Predictive Analytics Software for Windows, version 22, if not specified. Results were considered statistically significant if at or below .05 probability level.

FINDINGS

The descriptive statistics and bivariate correlations among the variables are shown in Table 1. All subscales and the overall scores of the Chinese Positive Youth Development Scale were significantly correlated ($r = .39$ to .63, $p < .01$). All subscales and the overall scores of the Chinese Family Assessment Instrument were significantly correlated ($r = .45$ to .59, $p < .01$). Analysis based on Pearson correlation showed that all CPYD and CFAI subscales were negatively correlated with the overall intentional and unintentional exposure to pornography ($r = -.03$ to -.13, $p < .01$), except for self-efficacy and resilience. Overall, higher levels of CPYD and CFAI were linked to lower levels of both types of exposure to pornography ($r = -.07$ to -.15, $p < .01$). Intentional exposure to pornography was positively correlated with unintentional exposure to pornography ($r = .54$, $p < .01$).

To further examine the impacts of individual and family background characteristics (i.e., CPYDS and CFAI) on both types of exposure to different kinds of pornographic materials, multiple regression analyses were used. In these models, intentional and unintentional exposures to different types of pornographic materials were regressed on the individual and family factors. The findings based on regression analyses are shown in tables 2-5.

Regarding the predictive effects of positive youth development, spirituality was a significant predictor of intentional exposure to pornographic video (β = -.08, $p < .05$), unintentional exposure to pornographic stories (β = -.10, $p < .01$) and pictures (β = -.07, $p < .05$). Social competence was a significant predictor of both types of exposure to pornographic pictures (unintentional: β = -.11, $p < .01$; intentional: β = -.10, $p < .01$). Resilience was a significant predictor of unintentional exposure to pornographic advertisements (β = -.09, $p < .05$). Results showed that higher levels of these exposures were found in individuals with lower levels of spirituality, social and moral competencies (Tables 2 and 3).

Table 2. The predictive effects of positive youth development on unintentional exposure to online pornography

unintentional						
	Stories	Pictures	Video	Chat room	Advertisement	Website
Predictor	β^a	β^a	β^a	β^a	β^a	β^a
BO	-.02	-.01	-.04	.003	-.05	-.01
RE	.03	.01	-.05	.02	-.09*	-.05
SC	-.07	-.11**	-.01	.01	.06	-.02
PB	-.01	-.01	-.02	-.03	-.003	-.03
EC	.05	.01	-.03	.02	-.03	-.07
MC	-.07	-.02	-.02	-.03	-.08*	-.02
SP	-.10**	-.07*	-.03	-.02	.03	.04
SE	.05	-.02	.03	-.02	.05	.05
R	.14	.17	.13	.06	.14	.11
R^2	.02	.03	.02	.00	.02	.01

Note: BO: bonding; RE: resilience; SC: social competence; PB: recognition for positive behavior; EC: emotional competence; MC: moral competence; SD: self-determination; SP: spirituality; SE: self-efficacy; $p < .05$*, $p < .01$**.

Table 3. The predictive effects of positive youth development on intentional exposure to online pornography

intentional						
	Stories	Pictures	Video	Chat room	Advertisement	Website
Predictor	β[a]	β[a]	β[a]	β[a]	β[a]	β[a]
BO	-.01	.02	-.02	.02	-.01	.01
RE	.03	-.01	-.01	-.001	-.02	-.02
SC	-.02	-.10**	-.01	-.02	.03	.02
PB	-.04	.02	-.03	-.01	-.03	-.07
EC	.01	.002	.01	.01	-.02	-.05
MC	-.06	-.06	-.05	.03	.003	-.02
SP	-.05	-.03	-.08*	-.05	.01	.01
SE	.02	.02	.04	-.07	-.04	.04
R	.09	.13	.12	.08	.06	.09
R^2	.01	.02	.02	.01	.004	.01

Note: BO: bonding; RE: resilience; SC: social competence; PB: recognition for positive behavior; EC: emotional competence; MC: moral competence; SD: self-determination; SP: spirituality; SE: self-efficacy; $p < .05$*, $p < .01$**.

Table 4. The predictive effects of family functioning on unintentional exposure to online pornography

unintentional						
	Stories	Pictures	Video	Chat room	Adverti-sement	Website
Predictor	β[a]	β[a]	β[a]	β[a]	β[a]	β[a]
Mutuality	-.04	-.07	-.17**	-.08	.01	-.12**
Harmony	-.003	-.03	-.03	.08*	.01	-.02
Communication	.02	-.03	.05	-.003	-.08*	.05
R	.07	.11	.16	.07	.07	.11
R^2	.01	.01	.03	.01	.01	.01

Note: $p < .05$*, $p < .01$** [a] standardized coefficients.

Among the constructs of family functioning, family mutuality had significant effects on two types of unintentional exposure to pornographic materials (video: $\beta = -.17, p < .01$; website: $\beta = -.12, p < .01$) and four types of intentional pornographic materials' exposures (video: $\beta = -.16, p < .01$; chat room: $\beta = -.14, p < .01$; advertisement: $\beta = -.16, p < .01$; website: β = -

.15, $p < .01$). Family communication significantly predicted changes in pornographic advertisements (unintentional: $\beta = -.08, p < .05$; intentional: $\beta = -.16$, $p < .01$) and pornographic websites (intentional: $\beta = -.10, p < .05$). Results revealed that individuals with higher levels of family mutuality and better communication displayed lower levels of these exposures (Tables 4 and 5).

In general, the overall score of CPYDS was a significant predictor of overall intentional and unintentional exposure to pornography. Positive youth development negatively predicted adolescents' unintentional ($\beta = -.12, p < .01$) and intentional exposure ($\beta = -.10, p < .01$) to pornography (see Table 6).

Table 5. The predictive effects of family functioning on intentional exposure to online pornography

intentional						
	Stories	Pictures	Video	Chat room	Adverti-sement	Website
Predictor	β^a	β^a	β^a	β^a	β^a	β^a
Mutuality	-.09	-.07	-.16**	-.14**	-.16**	-.15**
Harmony	.007	-.01	-.04	.05	.001	-.02
Communication	.07	.02	.07	.06	.16**	.10*
R	.06	.06	.14	.08	.11	.11
R^2	.003	.004	.02	.01	.01	.01

Note: $p < .05$*, $p < .01$** [a]standardized coefficients.

Table 6. The predictive effects of family functioning and positive youth development on two types of exposure to online pornography

	unintentional			intentional		
Predictor	R	R^2	β^a	R	R^2	β^a
PYD			-.12**			-.10**
CFAI			-.06			-.03
Model	.16	.03		.11	.01	

Note: PYD: total score of the positive youth development qualities; CFAI: total score of family functioning; [a] Standardized coefficients; $p < .05$*, $p < .01$**.

DISCUSSION

The purposes of the study were to explore the individual and family correlates of being exposed to online pornography and to compare the influence of these correlates on pornography exposure. The results of the study were summarized in three major findings.

First, as expected, greater positive youth development was associated with a decrease in both types of exposure to online pornography. Notably, several qualities of positive youth development (e.g., social competence and spirituality) were related to this outcome. People with good social competence usually have better quality social relationships. As previous studies have shown, the good quality of the social relationships was a significant predictor of a smaller likelihood of problematic behavior among adolescents in Slovakia (30), Hong Kong (14, 15) and the United States (6). Similarly, strong spirituality was related to fewer risky sexual behaviors (31-33). It seems that students who felt connected were less likely to be intentionally and unintentionally exposed to online pornography. Perhaps, the feeling of being attached to school or others result in a lower engagement in deviant behaviors (34, 35). The present findings extend the literature in exposure to online pornography.

Second, family functioning was related to a lower level of exposure to online pornography. The family is the primary social environment, which provides closeness and emotional support to the adolescents (36), that shapes adolescents' beliefs and attitudes towards sex. The present study demonstrated that family processes (i.e., mutuality and communication) play an important role in predicting adolescents' exposure to pornography, and thus, is in alignment with previous studies (8, 35, 36). This finding concurs with previous research that showed the positive family characteristics of frequent communication among family members and harmony reduced the likelihood of adolescents' problematic behaviors in the Western (38, 39) and Chinese context (14, 15).

Third, our analyses showed the protective effects of positive youth development and family functioning on both types of exposure to different online pornographic materials. Interestingly, positive youth development becomes the only significant predictor when examining the antecedents of both types of exposure to online pornography. This finding may be due to statistical artifact when composite scores of both factors were tested. Future research should adopt a structural equation model method in order to provide a meaningful examination of these antecedents on this behavior (40).

Although the present study is pioneering in its nature, several limitations should be noted. First, the majority of the participants were Hong Kong Chinese adolescents who were sampled from the general adolescent population. Therefore, the findings might not be generalizable to other populations. Second, other antecedents, such as peer influence was not tested in the present study. Peer influence has been found to be a significant predictor of adolescents' problematic behaviors, such as smoking (41) and sexual activity (42). The inclusion of peer influence might also improve the amount of variance explained when performing linear regression model analysis. Third, as the current data were based on one measurement time, future study should adopt a longitudinal design to examine the influence of these antecedents across time.

As a whole, with the easy availability and accessibility of the internet, adolescents are easily exposed to online pornography even if they do not have sexual intent. To protect them against this exposure, prevention efforts aiming at the family alone are not sufficient. Additional focus on the promotion of positive youth development is also necessary. The present study provides support for the influence of individual and family-related antecedents of adolescent's unintentional and intentional exposure to online pornography and sheds light on future youth intervention program.

ACKNOWLEDGMENTS

The present study is funded by a grant (Grant no. 25401414) of the Early Career Scheme of the Research Grants Council of the University Grants Committee of Hong Kong. The materials in this paper are based on a paper published in the *International Journal on Disability and Human Development* 2017;16(4) issue.

REFERENCES

[1] Shek DTL, Ma CMS. A six-year longitudinal study of consumption of pornographic materials in Chinese adolescents in Hong Kong. J Pediatr Adolesc Gynecol 2016;29(1):S12-21.

[2] Weber M, Quiring O, Daschmann G. Peers, parents and pornography: exploring adolescents' exposure to sexually explicit material and its developmental correlates. Sex Cult 2012;16(4):408-27.

[3] Hasking PA, Scheier LM, Abdallah AB. The three latent classes of adolescent delinquency and the risk factors for membership in each class. Aggress Behav 2011;37(1):19-35.

[4] Flood M. Exposure to pornography among youth in Australia. Aust NZ J Sociol 2007;43(1):45-60.

[5] Chen AS, Leung M, Chen CH, Yang SC. Exposure to internet pornography among Taiwanese adolescents. Soc Behav Pers 2013;41(1):157-64.

[6] Mesch GS. Social bonds and internet pornographic exposure among adolescents. J Adolesc 2009;32(3):601-18.

[7] Wolak J, Mitchell K, Finkelhor D. Unwanted and wanted exposure to online pornography in a national sample of youth Internet users. Pediatrics 2007;119(2):247-57.

[8] Ybarra ML, Mitchell KJ. Exposure to Internet pornography among children and adolescents: a national survey. Cyberpsychol Behav 2005;8(5):473-86.

[9] Doornwaard SM, van den Eijnden RJJM, Overbeek G, ter Bogt TFM. Differential developmental profiles of adolescents using sexually explicit internet material. J Sex Res 2015;52(3):269-81.

[10] Lo VH, Wei R. Exposure to internet pornography and Taiwanese adolescents' sexual attitudes and behavior. J Broadcast Electron Media 2005;49(2):221-37.

[11] Ybarra ML, Mitchell KJ, Hamburger M, Diener-West M, Leaf PJ. X-rated material and perpetration of sexually aggressive behavior among children and adolescents: Is there a link? Aggress Behav 2011;37(1):1-18.

[12] Morgan EM. Associations between young adults' use of sexually explicit materials and their sexual preferences, behaviors, and satisfaction. J Sex Res 2011;48(6):520-30.

[13] Peter J, Valkenburg PM. Adolescents' exposure to sexually explicit internet material and sexual satisfaction: a longitudinal study. Hum Commun Res 2009;35(2):171-94.

[14] Shek DTL, Ma CMS. Positive youth development and intention to gamble. In: Derevensky J, Shek DTL, Merrick J, eds. Adolescent Gambling. Berlin: de Gruyer, 2011.

[15] Shek DTL, Ma CMS. Substance abuse in junior secondary school students in Hong Kong: prevalence and psychosocial correlates. Int J Child Health Hum Dev 2011;4:433-42.

[16] Shek DTL. Positive youth development and behavioral intention to gamble among Chinese adolescents in Hong Kong. Int J Adolesc Med Health 2010;22(1):163-72.
[17] Shek DTL, Ma CMS, Tang CYP. Delinquency and problem behavior intention among early adolescents in Hong Kong: profiles and psychosocial correlates. Int J Disabil Hum Dev 2012;11(2):151-8.
[18] Sun RCF, Shek DTL. Life satisfaction, positive youth development, and problem behaviour among Chinese adolescents in Hong Kong. Soc Indic Res 2010;95(3):455-74.
[19] Shek DTL. A longitudinal study of perceived family functioning and adolescent adjustment in Chinese adolescents with economic disadvantage. J Fam Issues 2005;26(4):518-43.
[20] Elkington KS, Bauermeister JA, Zimmerman MA. Do parents and peers matter? a prospective socio-ecological examination of substance use and sexual risk among African American youth. J Adolesc 2011;34(5):1035-47.
[21] Wan GWY, Leung PWL. Factors accounting for youth suicide attempt in Hong Kong: a model building. J Adolesc 2010;33(5):575-82.
[22] Barrera M, Biglan A, Ary D, Li F. Replication of a problem behavior model with American Indian, Hispanic, and Caucasian youth. J Early Adolesc 2001;21(2):133-57.
[23] Engels RCME, Finkenauer C, van Kooten DC. Lying behavior, family functioning and adjustment in early adolescence. J Youth Adolesc 2006;35(6):949-58.
[24] Casey DM, Williams RJ, Mossière AM, Schopflocher DP, el-Guebaly N, Hodgins DC, et al. The role of family, religiosity, and behavior in adolescent gambling. J Adolesc 2011;34(5):841-51.
[25] Shek DTL, Ma CMS. Consumption of pornographic materials among Hong Kong early adolescents: a replication. ScientificWorldJournal 2012.
[26] Shek DTL, Ma CMS. Consumption of pornographic materials among early adolescents in Hong Kong: profiles and psychosocial correlates. Int J Disabil Hum Dev 2012;11(2):143-50.
[27] Ma CMS, Shek DTL. Consumption of pornographic materials in early adolescents in Hong Kong. J Pediatr Adolesc Gynecol 2013;26(3):S18-S25.
[28] Shek DT, Ma CM. Dimensionality of the Chinese positive youth development scale: confirmatory factor analyses. Soc Indic Res 2010;98:41-59.
[29] Shek DTL, Ma CMS. The Chinese family assessment instrument (C-FAI) hierarchical confirmatory factor analyses and factorial invariance. Res Soc Work Pract 2010;20(1):112-23.
[30] Kalina O, Geckova AM, Jarcuska P, Orosova O, Dijk JP, Reijneveld SA. Psychological and behavioural factors associated with sexual risk behaviour among Slovak students. BMC Public Health 2009;9(1):15-24.
[31] Chamratrithirong A, Miller BA, Byrnes HF, Rhucharoenpornpanich O, Cupp PK, Rosati MJ, et al. Spirituality within the family and the prevention of health risk

behavior among adolescents in Bangkok, Thailand. Soc Sci Med 2010;71(10):1855-63.

[32] Love SR. Illicit sexual behavior: a test of self-control theory. Deviant Behav 2006;27(5):505-36.

[33] O'Brien L-A, Denny S, Fleming T, Clark T, Teevale T, Robinson E. The impact of religion and spirituality on the risk behaviours of young people in aotearoa, New Zealand. Youth Stud Aust 2013;32(4).

[34] Cullen FT, Agnew R, Wilcox P. Criminological theory: past to present. New York: Oxford University Press, 2014.

[35] Wight D, Williamson L, Henderson M. Parental influences on young people's sexual behaviour: a longitudinal analysis. J Adolesc 2006;29(4):473-94.

[36] Ainsworth MDS. Object relations, dependency, and attachment: A theoretical review of the infant-mother relationship. Child Dev 1969:969-1025.

[37] Greenfield PM. Inadvertent exposure to pornography on the internet: implications of peer-to-peer file-sharing networks for child development and families. J Appl Dev Psychol 2004;25(6):741-50.

[38] Bersamin M, Todd M, Fisher DA, Hill DL, Grube JW, Walker S. Parenting practices and adolescent sexual behavior: a longitudinal study. J Marriage Fam 2008;70(1):97-112.

[39] Wellings K, Nanchahal K, Macdowall W, McManus S, Erens B, Mercer CH, et al. Sexual behaviour in Britain: early heterosexual experience. Lancet 2001;358 (9296):1843-50.

[40] Hancock GR, Lawrence FR, Nevitt J. Type I error and power of latent mean methods and MANOVA in factorially invariant and noninvariant latent variable systems. Struct Equ Modeling 2000;7(4):534-56.

[41] Poulin C, Graham L. The association between substance use, unplanned sexual intercourse and other sexual behaviours among adolescent students. Addiction 2001;96(4):607-21.

[42] Miller BC, Norton MC, Curtis T, Hill EJ, Schvaneveldt P, Young MH. The timing of sexual intercourse among adolescents family, peer, and other antecedents. Youth Soc 1997;29(1):54-83.

SECTION FOUR: LEADERSHIP

In: Soft Skills and Aspirations ...
Editors: Daniel TL Shek, et al.
ISBN: 978-1-53614-092-7

Chapter 12

QUALITATIVE EVALUATION OF A SERVICE LEADERSHIP SUBJECT IN A CHINESE CONTEXT

Daniel TL Shek[1-5,*], PhD, FHKPS, BBS, JP, Jing Wu[1], PhD, Li Lin[1], PhD and Emma XP Pu[1], PhD

[1]Department of Applied Social Sciences, The Hong Kong Polytechnic University, Hong Kong, PR China
[2]Centre for Innovative Programmes for Adolescents and Families, The Hong Kong Polytechnic University, Hong Kong, PR China
[3]Department of Social Work, East China Normal University, Shanghai, PR China
[4]Kiang Wu Nursing College of Macau, Macau, PR China
[5]Division of Adolescent Medicine, Department of Pediatrics, Kentucky Children's Hospital, University of Kentucky School of Medicine, Lexington, Kentucky, US

* Corresponding Author Email: daniel.shek@polyu.edu.hk.

ABSTRACT

Adopting a qualitative methodology, views of the students on a subject on Service Leadership were examined. Students taking the subject (N = 153) were invited to use descriptors and metaphors to describe their experiences about the subject. Regarding the descriptors given by the students, most of them were positive in nature. Similar positive findings were obtained for the metaphors. The findings are generally consistent with those studies using the same methodology reported in the literature. In conjunction with other evaluation findings, the present findings suggest that students had positive experiences about taking the subject and regarded the subject to be able to promote their service leadership qualities.

INTRODUCTION

Compared with manufacturing industries, service industries have taken an increasingly important role in most post-industrialized societies. As the economy structure shifts, desirable attributes of contemporary workers become quite different from those of workers in the past. Workers in the manufacturing economy were required to carry out repetitive tasks at the bottom layer of the decision-making pyramid (1). The key requirement for these workers was having technical skills only. On the contrary, workers in service economies are required to develop interpersonal and intrapersonal skills besides hard skills, such as communication skills, critical thinking, teamwork, work ethics, and self-management (2).

As the pillars of future society, graduates from tertiary institutions are expected to be proficient in both tangible hard skills and intangible soft skills. In fact, employers rated soft skills, such as communication, integrity, and flexibility, as fundamental factors for the success of an entry-level job (3). However, employers from all over the world also expressed their disappointment towards graduates about being lacking in communication, leadership, and management skills (4, 5). The Chief Human Resources Officer of CareerBuilder said that “One in five employers feel colleges do not adequately prepare students with crucial workplace competencies, including soft skills and real-world experience that might be gained through things like internships" (5). Therefore, to better prepare the students for entering the workforce, there is an urgent need for educators in tertiary institutions to emphasize soft skills education and to promote students' holistic development (6).

Among the highly desirable soft skills in the workplace, leadership has been recognized as one of the most valued generic graduate attributes in universities all over the world (7). In service economies, leadership structure is no longer highly top-down and autocratic, but rather open and autonomous (8). As a service-dominated society, the service sector shared 92.7% of the Gross Domestic Product (GDP) (9). There is a need to strengthen the service leadership and to maintain Hong Kong's competitiveness in the global market. To meet this need, Po Chung developed the service leadership model and founded The Hong Kong Institute of Service Leadership and Management (HKI-SLAM) in 2011 (10), where service leadership refers to "ethically satisfying the needs of self, others, groups, communities, systems, and environments" (11).

With the sponsorship of Victor and William Fung Foundation, the Service Leadership Initiative (SLI) in Hong Kong was launched with the participation of eight universities funded by the University Grants Committee (UGC), with each university incorporating the Service Leadership framework in their curricular and/or extra-curricular programs. At The Hong Kong Polytechnic University (PolyU), credit-bearing subjects and non-credit bearing programs have been successfully developed and implemented. Initially, a 2-credit Service Leadership subject was offered to students studying in the 3-year undergraduate program in the 2010/2013 academic years (12). Later on, a 3-credit CAR (Cluster Area Requirements) subject was developed and implemented since 2014/2015 academic year to students under 4-year curriculum. Besides, several intensive service leadership training programs jointly organized by PolyU and other universities in mainland China were also developed, including the "Global Youth Leadership Program" (GYLP) and the "Silk Road Youth Leadership Program" (SRYLP).

There are several rationales for developing Service Leadership subjects. First, in societies undergoing a rapid economic transformation, it is not surprising that the requirements for higher education have also been changing. Traditional leadership programs in universities are mostly aimed for "elitists" with the assumption that not everyone can be a leader (13). However, in a service-oriented society, all individuals are valuable human assets and inherent leaders. In an era of knowledge, complicated and multidisciplinary decision-making processes call for communication, sharing, and collaboration among multiple stakeholders. Human capital has become even more important than the tangible technologies.

Second, the existing leadership programs are largely concerned about interpersonal leadership competencies and rarely emphasize intrapersonal attributes (14). In comparison, the service leadership model proposed that effective service leaders should be excellent in not only competencies (e.g., task competency), but also in moral character (e.g., trustworthiness) and caring dispositions (e.g., sincerity and empathy). A study conducted by the Commission on Youth (15) showed 20% to 30% of adolescents in Hong Kong had strong materialistic orientations based on wealth and hedonism. Therefore, it is imperative to deliver moral education among adolescents through conducting service leadership education (16).

Third, given the intensification of adolescent developmental problems (such as substance abuse, lifestyle issues, and mental disorders), youths in Hong Kong are easily get lost without proper career and life guidance (17, 18). From an ecological perspective, Service Leadership courses can help prevent adolescent problem behaviors at both an individual level (such as promoting social-emotional competencies) and environmental level (such as fostering bonding and sense of social responsibility). In general, the Service Leadership subjects promote the whole-person development of university students in Hong Kong (19, 20).

The 3-credit General Education subject entitled "Service Leadership" was developed to help university students: "1) learn the basic models of leadership with respect to the service sector and compare their assertions, strengths, and weaknesses; 2) understand the basic leadership attributes intrinsic to effective service leaders, including leadership competencies, moral character, and caring dispositions; 3) reflect on their own service leadership qualities, including leadership competencies, moral character, and caring disposition; 4) learn to develop and apply the basic qualities of an effective service leader; 5) cultivate an appreciation of the importance of Service Leadership to the development and wellness of oneself, other people and the whole society" (21).

To demonstrate the accountability, outcomes, and impacts of the Service Leadership subjects, systematic evaluation was conducted for every class. Both quantitative (i.e., one-group pre-test/post-test pre-experimental design, objective outcome evaluation, and subjective outcome evaluation) and qualitative (i.e., focus groups, and reflection sheet) methods were employed. The dominance of quantitative orientation in educational research began since the movement toward a "scientific method of education" (22). The equal emphasis of qualitative research has not been recognized till the early 1980s. Though the quantitative approach is superior in generalizability relying on large samples, the qualitative approach also has its strength that captures an in-depth understanding of complicated information with a small sample, such as students' deep feelings and reflections (23). Besides, the design of qualitative studies is more flexible and personalized, such as the use of follow-up questions based on participants' responses during an interview (24). Furthermore, qualitative research has its advantage in eliciting unexpected findings (25).

As a matter of fact, rather than using either single method, a combination of quantitative and qualitative evaluation is always much more effective (26). The previous studies have provided a comprehensive evaluation of the Service Leadership subject in its first two years' implementation (27-33). For example, the results of data collected from 60 students in the 2012/2013 academic year showed that after taking the Service Leadership subject, students had positive changes in the areas of moral competence, behavioral competence, character strengths, general positive youth development qualities, and overall service leadership qualities (29). In the present study, students' responses to the reflection sheets were analyzed to evaluate the Service Leadership subject from a qualitative perspective. In this study, students were invited to use three "descriptors" and one "metaphor" to describe their experiences about the subject. A similar method was used in the 2012/2013 academic year. Based on 50 students who participated in the study, results showed that 96.1% of the descriptors and 90% of the metaphors used by students were positive ones (28). In this study, the data collected in 2014/2015 academic year were reported.

OUR STUDY

We invited all the students who took the subject “Service leadership” in Semester 1 and 2 of the academic year of 2014/2015 to write down their personal reflections on this course. Students were informed about the confidentiality of their responses at the beginning. They were also notified that they could withdraw from this study without any punishment. Student individual consent was collected before data collection. Students were asked to write down three words or phrases (i.e., descriptors) to describe their experiences, perceptions or feelings of the learning experience (e.g., “interesting”). They were also required to think about an object, an event, or a state (i.e., metaphors) to stand for the course (e.g., “enjoyable tour”). To ensure that we can really understand the metaphors that students used, they were required to give a brief explanation of the meaning of the metaphors they used. For example, one student indicated that “Ocean Park” could stand for his/her impression of the course, and then he/she wrote “just like Ocean Park, this course includes lots of content for us and every time I come in the classroom, I experience different feelings including inspiration and excitement.” A total of 85 students in Semester 1 and 68 students in Semester 2 completed and submitted their reflection sheets after the completion of the course. The response rates were 88.5% and 85.0%, respectively.

Data analyses

The responses in the reflection sheets were transcribed and coded. The coders were two research staff who did not participate in the data collection. Since the unit of analysis in the current study was a meaningful unit instead of a statement, if two words with different meanings were mentioned in one phrase, the phrase would be divided into two meaningful units. For example, the statement that this course was "enjoyable and useful" would be broken down into two meaningful units: "enjoyable" and "useful". On the other hand, different descriptions with the similar meaning (e.g., "interesting" and "fun") were grouped into one meaningful unit. This practice was applied to both descriptors and metaphors. The current coding system was adopted in previous studies (17, 34, 35). After initial coding, the descriptors or metaphors were classified into four categories (positive, negative, neutral, and undecided). To test intra- and inter-rater reliability, 20 descriptors and 20 metaphors for each semester were randomly selected from the raw response. For the intra-rater reliability, two research staffs who were involved in the coding process recoded these randomly selected raw responses, while for inter-rater reliability, two other research staff, which did not participate in initial coding, were asked to code these randomly selected raw responses independently.

FINDINGS

Table 1 and Table 2 show the raw descriptors and their categories in Semester 1 and Semester 2 of the academic year of 2014/2015, respectively. According to Table 1 (Semester 1), 96.89% ($n = 249$) of the descriptors were positive ones. The category of "interesting/fun" ($n = 36$) comprised the largest proportion of positive descriptors. Only one neutral descriptor (0.39%, "different") was recorded. 1.56% ($n = 4$) could be regarded as negative descriptors, such as "boring" and "difficult". Three undecided descriptors (1.17%) were recorded, which were "challenging", "high EQ" and "unexpected". Similar findings were observed in Table 2 (Semester 2), where 95.63% ($n = 197$) could be classified as positive descriptors, such as "inspiring" and "relax". The category of "interesting/fun" ($n = 29$) was the most frequently mentioned positive descriptors; 2.43% ($n = 5$) could be regarded as neutral descriptors, such as "change" and "discussion". Three negative descriptors (1.46%) were recorded, which were "frustrated", "complicated" and "talkative", whereas only one undecided descriptor (0.49%, "servant") was recorded. In sum, for both semesters, positive feedback comprised the biggest share of all feedback. Students generally gave positive feedback in descriptors, such "interesting/fun", "useful", and "inspiring/encourage". We also adopted the chi-square test to explore the difference of descriptors between Semester 1 and Semester 2. The result indicated that no difference between Semester 1 and Semester 2 was observed, $\chi^2_{(3)} = 4.54$, $p = .21$. For the descriptors, the intra-rater agreement reached 100% for both research staff in both semesters. The inter-rater agreement percentages calculated between every two researchers was 80% in Semester 1 and ranged from 80% to 90% in Semester 2. This indicated that the codes given by different researchers were highly consistent.

For metaphors in Semester 1 (see Table 3), 85 raw metaphors were classified into positive, neutral, negative, and undecided responses. As shown in Table 3 (Semester 1), all raw metaphors (100%) were seen as positive responses, such as "key", "map", and "guiding light", while no metaphor was regarded as neutral, negative or undecided. The result of Semester 2 (Table 4) was similar to the result of Semester 1, among 67 raw metaphors, 98.33% ($n = 66$) could be seen as positive metaphors, such as "meaningful journey", "light bulb", and "water", whereas 1.49% ($n = 1$) could be seen as neutral metaphors, which was "roller coaster". No metaphor was seen as negative or undecided. The chi-square test was also used to explore the difference of metaphors between Semester 1 and Semester 2. The result revealed that there was no difference between Semester 1 and Semester 2, $\chi^2_{(1)} = .01$, $p = .91$. The intra-rater agreement reached 95% for both research staff in Semester 1, while it reached 95% and 100% respectively for the two research staff in Semester 2. The inter-rater agreement percentages calculated between every two researchers ranged from 90% to 100% in Semester 1 and 85% to 90% in Semester 2, suggesting there was high reliability in the coding.

The metaphors used by students were various. According to Table 3 and Table 4, the most frequently mentioned metaphors included "journey", "light bulb", "guideline", and "compass in life". Here we listed some examples of students' typical positive metaphors and their illustrations:

Table 1. Categorization of descriptors used by the participants to describe the course in Semester 1 of the academic year of 2014/2015

Descriptors	Nature of the Response				Total
	Positive	Neutral	Negative	Undecided	
Interesting/fun	36				
Helpful/helpful in self-reflection/helpful in personal growth	29				
Inspiring/encouraging	26				
Useful/practical/useful for Development	20				
Meaningful	20				
Interactive	16				
Knowledgeable/informative	14				
Improving leadership	9				
Stimulating	8				
Creative	7				
Share/communication	7				
Amazing/memorable	6				
Reality	6				
Happy	6				
Caring	5				
Making self-reflection	5				
Relaxing/refreshing	4				
Fruitful	4				
Open minded	3				
Nice	3				
Others positive responses	15				
Different		1			
Boring			2		
Difficult			2		
Challenging				1	
High EQ				1	
Unexpected				1	
Total Count (N):	249	1	4	3	257
Total Count (%):	96.89%	.39%	1.56%	1.17%	100.00 %

Note: Other positive responses included the positive descriptors once or twice.

Table 2. Categorization of descriptors used by the participants to describe the course in Semester 2 of the academic year of 2014/2015

Descriptors	Nature of the Response				Total
	Positive	Neutral	Negative	Undecided	
Interesting/fun	29				
Useful	18				
Inspiring/encourage	11				
Good/amazing/wonderful	10				
Happy/joyful	9				
Service leadership	9				
Helpful	8				
Meaningful	8				
Practical	6				
Interaction	6				
Relax	5				
Reflection	5				
Intrapersonal	5				
Valuable	4				
Studying/learning	4				
Unforgettable/memorable	4				
Enjoy	3				
Creative	3				
Future	3				
Interpersonal	3				
Excited	3				
Enlightening/educational	3				
Wisdom	3				
Active/motivational	3				
Attractive	3				
Acknowledge	3				
Others positive responses	26				
New		1			
Discussion		1			
Change		1			
Activities		1			
Unexpected		1			
Frustrated			1		
Complicated			1		
Talkative			1		
Servant				1	
Total Count (N):	197	5	3	1	206
Total Count (%):	95.63%	2.43%	1.46%	0.49%	100.00%

Note: Other positive responses included the positive descriptors once or twice.

Table 3. Categorization of the metaphors used by the participants to describe the course in Semester 1 of the academic year of 2014/2015

Metaphors	Nature of the Metaphor					Number of Codes Derived from the Metaphor and Its Nature				
	Positive	Neutral	Negative	Undecided	Total	Positive	Neutral	Negative	Undecided	Total
Light bulb/lighted candle/candle/a bright lamp/flashlight/streetlight/guiding light/light	11					18	1			
Traveling/travel/enlightening journey/in-depth exploration journey/enjoyable tour/training camp	9					17				
Compass in life	5					9				
Apple tree/tree	3					7				
Guide map/map	3					5				
Cooking book/a book called service leadership/book	3					3				
Buffet	3					3	1			
Other positive responses (e.g., life coach, encyclopedia, gift)	48					88	5			
Total Count (N):	85	0	0	0	85	150	7	0	0	157
Total Count (%):	100%				100%	95.54%	4.46%			100%

Note: Other positive responses included the positive metaphors reported less than thrice.

Table 4. Categorization of the metaphors used by the participants to describe the course in Semester 2 of the academic year of 2014/2015

Metaphors	Nature of the Metaphor					Number of Codes Derived from the Metaphor and Its Nature				
	Positive	Neutral	Negative	Undecided	Total	Positive	Neutral	Negative	Undecided	Total
Meaningful journey/fantastic journey/ special journey/journey/big bus tour/museum tour/enjoyable tour/road trip/trip/long travel	13					24				
Light bulb/bulb/light/candle/lamp	6					11				
Buffet	3					5				
A cup filled with water/water	3					4				
Other positive responses (e.g., lollipop moment, rainbow, wings)	41					73	1			
Roller coaster		1				1		1		
Total Count (N):	66	1	0		67	118	1	1		120
Total Count (%):	98.51%	1.49%			100%	98.33%	0.83%	0.83%		100%

- "*Meaningful journey*": "through the lectures, I have known more about the characteristic of being an effective service leader. Besides, this course can help me enhance the sense of being an all dimension (holistic) leader."
- "*Compass in life*": "it teaches you about the skills of how to be with the others harmoniously, as well as you will know what the modern leadership should be, you will be able to catch up territory there."
- "*Lamp*": "the course reveals how to be an effective service leader, just like the lamp that can lead me to the brightness. After this course, I hope I can be competent, ethical and caring."
- "*Map*": "The course suggests a new way of leadership which is service leadership. It gives me one more direction to apply the leadership style in my own hospitality industry."
- "*Training camp*": "the course divides students into several groups and students need to deal with people with from different backgrounds and work together. This helps to enhance their communication and leadership skills, and finally establish team spirit as well as friendship."
- "*Buffet*": "the course has many different aspects of knowledge regarding the service leadership. Also, the format of the lessons is multiple, include lecture, interactive activities, communication."

According to Table 3 and Table 4, only a few sentences of the explanations were seen as neutral or negative responses. In some cases, even if the explanation was neutral, the metaphor was still seen as a positive response. For example, one student who used "water" as the metaphor said that "*this course's information seems to be simple, but it is essential to our growth.*" The first sentence "*this course's information seems to be simple*" was coded as a neutral response, while the second sentence "*but it is essential to our growth*" was regarded as a positive response. Therefore, the metaphor "water" was still regarded as a positive response. In all, students generally hold positive feedback towards this course.

DISCUSSION

The present study investigated the effectiveness of the "Service leadership" subject at The Hong Kong Polytechnic University in the 2014/2015 academic year. A qualitative approach was employed to explore students' perceptions and feelings towards the subject. Consistent with our expectations, the dominant view was positive that over ninety percent (96.89% in Semester 1 and 95.63% in Semester 2) of the students listed positive descriptors to express their impression on the courses in both semesters. Likewise, almost all students (100% in Semester 1 and 98.33% in Semester 2) used positive metaphors to reflect their cognitive and emotional understandings of the learning processes in the Service Leadership subject. The findings are consistent with the existing qualitative evaluation studies on both credit-bearing Service Leadership subject and non-credit-bearing programs (e.g., 35, 36). In general, the subject was described as "good/amazing/wonderful", "unforgettable/memorable", "attractive", "fruitful", and "meaningful". Besides, the prevailing metaphors students used are "Journey/traveling/trip/tour/camp", such as "in-depth exploration journey", "museum tour", "training camp", and "fantastic journey". There were several types of evidence suggesting that the Service Leadership subject is effective in promoting the holistic development of the students.

Most of the positive descriptors were expressed from an instrumental perspective. Students described the subject as "useful", "helpful in self-reflection/helpful in personal growth", "knowledgeable", "practical". Correspondingly, the utility value was also seen in many metaphors, such as "light bulb/lighted candle", "life coach/encyclopedia", "compass in life", and "guide map/cooking book". One of the leading purposes of implementing the Service Leadership subject is to promote students' self-reflecting ability. Hence, it is delightful that the Service Leadership subject could achieve the purpose of strengthening students' awareness of self-reflection, self-understanding, as well as self-development.

The second most positive descriptors were related to the positive emotions of the students. The Service Leadership subject was perceived as "interesting/fun", "happy/joyful", "relaxing", "excited", and "refreshing". Expressions about happiness also emerged in the metaphors, such as "enjoyable tour", and "lollipop moment". All these emotional descriptors and metaphors indicated that the subject provided an enjoyable and inspiring learning experience. During the classes, students gained knowledge, ability, and happiness at the same time.

In the current study, students across semesters also expressed their appreciation towards the teaching and learning styles using descriptors like "interaction", "reflection", "active/motivational", "creative", and "share/ communication". The Service Leadership subject has been characterized by its interactive and experience-based teaching and learning methods. The paradigm shift from passive learning to active learning promotes students' engagement in classes and promotes their life-long learning ability (37, 38).

Although the findings in the present study were remarkably positive, there were still several negative perceptions (four in Semester 1 and three in Semester 2) on the subject. Taking the descriptors in Semester 1 as an example, two students described the subject as "difficult" and another two described it as "boring". Although the negative comments were in the minority, it is important to understand why some students had such negative views in future.

The current study showed several strengths of qualitative methods in program evaluation. First, students encapsulated their abstract and complex feelings and experiences during the Service Leadership courses into direct and cohesive descriptors and metaphors (39). Particularly, unlike other research methods that rely on established mental sets when designing research questions, metaphors allowed participants more freedom to use their creativity to reflect on specific opinions. Secondly, it is a vivid way to gather abundant information from the informants' perspectives that researchers or practitioners have not considered or expected in advance. Lastly, qualitative evaluation is helpful to further improve the program by pointing out some negative responses (35).

Several limitations of the study should also be highlighted. Primarily, as mentioned above, the descriptors and metaphors can be used to reduce the complexity of heterogeneous pieces of information. However, "highlighting" also brings about "hiding". The interpretation of the forced-simplified descriptors and metaphors has high demands for researchers' discriminatory ability (40). To better elaborate the descriptors and metaphors and to verify the interpretations, further in-depth interviews should be conducted, including individual interviews and focus groups. Besides, the reflection sheets were collected only at one time point, which cannot represent the dynamic quality of the implementation of the Service Leadership subject. It would be more convincing if qualitative studies at multiple time points could be conducted. Finally, the validity of the qualitative evaluations mostly depends on the researchers' knowledge, training, and practices (41). Therefore, peer-checking and member-checking would improve the truthful understanding of the effectiveness evaluation, which are advocated in future studies.

Despite the aforementioned limitations, the findings of the present study provide continuous supportive evidence for the positive nature of the Service Leadership subject and the effectiveness of its implementation during the 2014/2015 academic year.

ACKNOWLEDGMENTS

The Service Leadership Education project at The Hong Kong Polytechnic University was financially supported by the Victor and William Fung Foundation. The materials in this chapter are based on a paper published in the *International Journal on Disability and Human Development* 2017;16(4) issue.

REFERENCES

[1] Wilhelm WJ. Research on workplace skills employers want. In: Meeting the demand: Teaching "soft" skills. Delta Pi Epsilon Society, Little Rock, AR, 2002:12-33.

[2] Sorenson G. An intellectual history of leadership studies: The role of James MacGregor Burns. Washington, DC: American Political Science Association, 2002.

[3] Weber MR, Finley DA, Crawford A, Rivera D. An exploratory study identifying soft skill competencies in entry-level managers. Tour Hosp Res 2009;9(4):353-61.

[4] British Association of Graduate Recruiters, AGR. Low wages not education to blame for skills gap, says University of Warwick. URL: https://warwick.ac.uk/newsandevents/news/low_wages_not/

[5] CareerBuilder. Companies planning to hire more recent college graduates this year and pay them better, according to CareerBuilder survey. URL: http://www.careerbuilder.com/share/aboutus/pressreleasesdetail.aspx?sd=4%2F23%2F2015&id=pr889&ed=12%2F31%2F2015.

[6] Tempone I, Kavanagh M, Segal N, Hancock P, Howieson B, Kent J. Desirable generic attributes for accounting graduates into the twenty-first century: The views of employers. Accout Res J 2012;25(1):41-55.

[7] Ewing JC, Bruce JA, Ricketts KG. Effective leadership development for undergraduates: How important is active participation in collegiate organizations. J Leadersh Educ 2009;7(3):118-32.

[8] Uhl-Bien M, Marion R, McKelvey B. Complexity leadership theory: Shifting leadership from the industrial age to the knowledge era. Leadersh Q 2007;18(4):298-318.

[9] The World Bank. Services, etc., value added (% of GDP). URL: http://data.worldbank.org/indicator/NV.SRV.TETC.ZS/

[10] Chung PPY. Service leadership definitions. URL: http://hki-slam.org/index.php?r=article&catid=1&aid=11.

[11] Chung PPY. Hong Kong Institute of Service Leadership and Management (SLAM) curriculum framework. Hong Kong: Hong Kong institute of leadership and management, 2011. Available at: http://hki-slam.org/index.php?r=article&catid=3&aid=38.

[12] Shek DTL, Yu L, Ma CMS, Sun RCF, Liu TT. Development of a credit-bearing service leadership subject for university students in Hong Kong. Int J Adolesc Med Health 2013;25(4):353-61.

[13] Layfield KD, Radhakrishna RB, Andreasen RJ. Self-perceived leadership skills of students in a leadership programs in agriculture course. J Agric Educ Res 2000;50(1):62-8.

[14] Shek DTL, Lin L, Liu TT. Service leadership education for university students in Hong Kong: Subjective outcome evaluation. Int J Disabil Hum Dev 2014;13(4):513-21.

[15] Commission on Youth. Study on Civic Awareness and Moral Values of Youth, Government of the Hong Kong Special Administrative Region, Hong Kong, 2000.

[16] Shek DTL, Ma CMS, Lin L. The Chinese adolescent materialism scale: psychometric properties and normative profiles. Int J Disabil Human Dev 2014;13(2):285-95.

[17] Shek DTL. Adolescent developmental issues in Hong Kong: relevance to positive youth development programs in Hong Kong. Int J Adolesc Med Health 2006;18(3):341-54.

[18] Shek DTL, Keung MH, Sun RCF. A brief overview of adolescent developmental problems in Hong Kong. ScientificWorldJournal 2011;11:2243-56.
[19] Shek DTL. Nurturing holistic development of university students in Hong Kong: where are we and where should we go?. ScientificWorldJournal 2010;10:563-75.
[20] Shek DTL, Sun RCF, Chui YH, Lit SW, Yuen WW, Chung YYH, Ngai SW. Development and evaluation of a positive youth development course for university students in Hong Kong. ScientificWorldJournal 2012. DOI: 10.1100/2012/263731.
[21] Shek DTL. Course outline for service leadership. Hong Kong: The Hong Kong Polytechnic University, 2015.
[22] Cronbach LJ, Suppes P. Research for tomorrow's schools: Disciplined inquiry for education. London: Macmillan, 1969.
[23] Shulman LS. Disciplines of inquiry in education: an overview. Educ Res 1981;10(6):5-12.
[24] Turner III DW. Qualitative interview design: A practical guide for novice investigators. Qual Rep 2010;15(3):754-60.
[25] Bryman A. Integrating quantitative and qualitative research: how is it done? Qual Res 2006;6(1):97-113.
[26] Snape D, Spencer L. The foundations of qualitative research. In: Ritchie J, Lewis J, Nicholls CM, Ormston R, eds. Qualitative research practice: A guide for social science students and researchers. Thousand Oaks, CA: Sage, 2003:1-23.
[27] Shek DTL, Li X. Evaluation of an innovative leadership training program for Chinese students: Subjective outcome evaluation. Int J Disabil Hum Dev 2015;14(4):393-400.
[28] Shek DTL, Lin L, Liu TT. Service leadership education for university students in Hong Kong: Subjective outcome evaluation. Int J Disabil Hum Dev 2014;13(4):513-21.
[29] Shek DTL, Yu L, Ma CMS. The students were happy but did they change positively? Yes, they did. Int J Disabil Hum Dev 2014;13(4):505-11.
[30] Shek DTL, Law MYM, Liu TT. Focus group evaluation of a service leadership subject in Hong Kong. Int J Disabil Hum Dev 2015;14(4):371-6.
[31] Shek DTL, Sun RCF. Promoting psychosocial competencies in university students: Evaluation based on a one-group pre-test/post-test design. Int J Disabil Hum Dev 2012;11(3):229-34.
[32] Shek DTL, Ma CMS. Do university students change after taking a subject on leadership and intrapersonal development? Int J Disabil Hum Dev 2014;13(4):451-6.
[33] Shek DTL, Lin L. Changes in university students after joining a service leadership program in China. J Leadersh Educ 2016;15(1):96-109.
[34] Shek DTL, Ng CSM. Qualitative evaluation of the Project PATHS: Findings based on focus groups with student participants. ScientificWorldJournal 2009;9:691-703.
[35] Shek DTL, Sun RCF. Qualitative evaluation of a positive youth development course in a university setting in Hong Kong. Int J Disabil Hum Dev 2012;11(3):243-48.
[36] Shek DTL, Lin L. Service leadership education in the global youth leadership programme: A qualitative evaluation. Int J Child Adolesc Health 2016;9(2):245-52.

[37] Bryson C, Hand L. The role of engagement in inspiring teaching and learning. Innov Educ Teach Int 2007;44(4):349-62.

[38] Garvin MR, Ramsier RD. Experiential learning at the university level: A US case study. Educ Train 2003;45(5):280-5.

[39] Cade BW. Some uses of metaphor. Aust J Fam Ther 1982;3(3):135-40.

[40] Schmitt R. Systematic metaphor analysis as a method of qualitative research. Qual Rep 2005;10(2):358-94.

[41] Shek DTL, Tang V, Han XY. Evaluation of Evaluation Studies Using Qualitative Research Methods in the Social Work Literature (1990-2003): Evidence That Constitutes a Wake-Up Call. Res Soc Work Pract 2005;15 (3):180-94.

In: Soft Skills and Aspirations …
Editors: Daniel TL Shek, et al.
ISBN: 978-1-53614-092-7

Chapter 13

CHINESE STUDENTS IN HONG KONG AND THEIR VIEW ON GENERAL EDUCATION

Daniel TL Shek*[1-6,*]*, PhD, FHKPS, BBS, SBS, JP,
Florence KY Wu*[1]*, EdD and Wen Yu Chai*[1]*, PhD
[1]Department of Applied Social Sciences,
The Hong Kong Polytechnic University, Hong Kong, PR China
[2]Center for Innovative Programmes for Adolescents and Families,
The Hong Kong Polytechnic University, Hong Kong, PR China
[3]Department of Social Work, East China Normal University,
Shanghai, PR China
[4]Kiang Wu Nursing College of Macau, Macau, PR China
[5]Hong Kong Institute of Service Leadership and Management,
Hong Kong, PR China
[6]Division of Adolescent Medicine, Kentucky Children's Hospital,
University of Kentucky, Lexington, Kentucky, US

* Corresponding Author Email: daniel.shek@polyu.edu.hk.

ABSTRACT

The General University Requirements (GUR) is a component of the new 4-year undergraduate program at The Hong Kong Polytechnic University. This study examined students' views and experiences of the GUR using a qualitative methodology. Written comments of 240 freshmen, sophomores, and senior-year students with reference to open-ended questions on their memorable experiences in GUR study were collected. The qualitative findings suggested that students generally had positive views of the GUR in terms of its widely-adopted active and experiential learning pedagogy, useful and attractive contents, caring teaching staff, and rich learning outcomes. Challenges were also identified for further improvement of the GUR.

INTRODUCTION

Historically, general education has been an essential part of American college education. It is a common education for all undergraduates aiming to offer students a broad exposure to different knowledge disciplines and nurture the intellectual and civic attributes of students (1). For many centuries, the value of general education was constantly claimed and regarded as more significant in contemporary society. Along with the development of science and technology, as well as increased specialization of knowledge since the twentieth century, general education becomes more important since it is a good counter-measure to overspecialization of knowledge through providing students a common body of knowledge and intellectual experiences (2, 3). In another word, general education is vital to prevent disconnections and disunity in students' learning (4). As argued by Boyer and Levine (5), "overspecialization, excessive vocationalism, and above all, the free-elective system were criticized for ignoring the broad purposes of education. General education, it was argued, would help restore the balance" (p. 30). Also, McGrath (6), one former editor of *The Journal of General Education* claimed that general education was "the unifying element of a culture. It embraces the great moral truths, the scientific generalizations, the aesthetic conceptions, and the spiritual values of the race, ignorance of which makes men incapable of understanding themselves and the world in which they live" (p. 3).

In modern societies, general education also assumes the task of helping students develop to be effective and functional citizens to tackle complicated problems that are hard to be solved by knowledge from one discipline (7). With the emergence of globalized knowledge economies, there are increasing insecurity and instability in career development for university graduates. Hence, nurturing university students to be flexible and have transferrable generic skills to succeed in the society is an important task for university educators (2, 8). Against this background, more and more governments acknowledged the importance of general education in their manpower development and incorporated general education programs into curricula of their higher education (9). In the United States, the value of general education has also been reclaimed as an important strategy for empowering university students to compete in a global and multicultural society (10).

General education has also been rigorously introduced into the undergraduate curriculum of the Hong Kong higher education system. Before the handover back to China in 1997, Hong Kong had developed a higher education tradition that inherited the structure of British higher education. Its undergraduate degree program was featured by a three-year curriculum with early specialization in students (11). In this structure, general education only occupied a marginalized place. However, Hong Kong carried out a reform on its higher education system after the handover to transfer its three-year British style of higher education to four-year American style of higher education. Commencing from the fall of 2012, mandated by the University Grants Committee (UGC), a government advisory committee for higher education funding and development, all eight public universities in Hong Kong changed their undergraduate degree programs. Specifically, the length of all three-year undergraduate degree programs was changed to four years. At the same time, a foundational general education component was introduced into the new four-year undergraduate curriculum in each university.

With specific reference to The Hong Kong Polytechnic University (PolyU), along with the transition from a three-year to a four-year structure of undergraduate education, PolyU developed a significant general education component named "General University Requirements" (GUR) in its new four-year curriculum. With its six featured components, the GUR aimed to nurture the graduates with five desired graduate attributes, including effective communication, critical thinking, innovative problem solving, lifelong learning, and ethical leadership. The six components of the GUR are as follows:

- Freshman Seminar (FS, 3 credits): FS is a mandatory subject for first year students. It is offered by each faculty/school to their students regardless of their specializations. It introduces students to their potential disciplines and majors.
- Leadership and Intra-personal Development (LIPD, 3 credits): LIPD component aims to develop students' interpersonal and intrapersonal qualities conducive to effective and ethical leadership. While students at the Faculty of Business take "Tango! Managing Self and Others" ("Tango!"), other students take a subject entitled "Tomorrow's Leaders" (TL).
- Language and Communication Requirements (LCR, 9 credits). LCR component aims to strengthen students' language proficiencies in both English and Chinese. In this component, all students are required to take two English subjects (6 credits) and one Chinese subject (3 credits).
- Cluster Area Requirements (CAR, 12 credits). CAR component aims to expose students to knowledge of different disciplines. It also tries to develop students' understanding of China and their reading and writing skills. In this component, students are required to take one elective subject from each of the four cluster areas of learning. The four cluster areas are: CAR-A "Human Nature, Relations and Development", CAR-B "Community, Organization and Globalization", CAR-C "History, Culture and World Views", and CAR-D "Science, Technology and Environment". Besides, students

also need to fulfill three additional requirements in the CAR subjects: (a) China Studies Requirements (CSR), (b) English Writing and Reading Requirements (EW/ER), and (c) Chinese Writing and Reading Requirements (CW/CR).

- Service Learning (SL, 3 credits). SL component aims to help students apply academic knowledge in solving real world problems, help them reflect on their roles as responsible citizens, and develop their empathy and civic responsibility.
- Healthy Lifestyle (HLS, non-credit-bearing). HLS component helps students to establish a healthy lifestyle. Students are required to complete a program with four components covering different dimensions of health: introductory lecture, sports training, e-learning, and wrap-up lecture.

A unique feature of the GUR is its active and experiential learning pedagogy embedded in different program components. For example, group project work is widely adopted as a major approach of student learning and assessment in subjects of different GUR components including FS, LIPD, CAR, and SL. Meanwhile, experiential learning occupies a significant component in subjects in SL and HLS components. In addition, the writing assignment is also adopted as a major mean of assessment in many subjects.

Although the value of general education and its benefits to student development have been proposed by different philosophers and educators for centuries, empirical studies on how students perceive general education and its effects on their development are not adequate. Some limited number of studies gives insights in this area. For example, Twombly (12) found that while some students perceived general education as helpful to their academic confidence, study habits, social network, and major selection, more students perceived a failed alignment of general education with its intended goals. Twombly (12, 13) found that students valued general education programs that were more related with their professional goals. King and Kotrlik (14) suggested that students preferred general education curricula that were broad and gave them more flexibility. Vander Schee (15) found that first-year seminar in general education that introduced students to their broad disciplines and university academic life had enhanced students' appreciation of general education program and their confidence in subject selection in general education. Some newly promoted curriculum mode in general education such as Service Learning was found to have high positive impact on student development in terms of critical thinking, writing skills, leadership, problem solving, interpersonal skills, and self-efficacy (16, 17). These studies suggested what curricula factors perceived by students as effective in promoting their positive learning in general education. Nevertheless, the available studies were based on the contexts of American higher education, which does not reflect students' views of general education in higher education in other cultural contexts.

Against this background, the present study investigated how students perceived the General University Requirements (GUR) in the new four-year curriculum of The Hong Kong Polytechnic University (PolyU) through collecting and analyzing the written responses of the students to open-ended questions. The present study was one component of a five-year longitudinal evaluation project starting from the 2012-2013 academic year, aiming to evaluate the implementation and effectiveness of the GUR at PolyU. The project comprised several major components, including objective outcome evaluation based on a four-year longitudinal online survey, subjective outcome evaluation based on student feedback questionnaires, qualitative evaluation based on student and teacher focus groups, and students and teachers' written responses to qualitative evaluation forms. The objective outcome evaluation findings revealed that students had significant positive changes on important inter- and intra-personal attributes (18, 19). The subjective outcome evaluation findings showed that GUR subjects were generally well-received by students and promoted students' learning experiences over time (20). Because these evaluation studies were based on quantitative methods, they could not show the subjective experiences of the students. Although focus group is a good method to collect students' views, it is more resource-consuming comparing to written responses because much time and manpower are required for focus group interviews and transcription tasks. Also, students' individual views could be influenced by their peers in focus group interactions. Therefore, analysis of individual written responses to open-ended questions is an alternative way to collect students' views in an efficient and objective manner. In this study, qualitative evaluation of the GUR based on students' written responses was carried out.

Table 1. Numbers of participants by faculty and cohort in GUR qualitative evaluation

Cohort	Faculty								
	FAST	FB	FCE	FENG	FH	FHSS	SD	SHTM	Total
2012-2013	9	7	5	11	10	9	4	9	64
2013-2014	12	11	14	13	12	10	10	5	87
2014-2015	15	8	9	10	12	12	9	14	89
Total	36	26	28	34	34	31	23	28	240

Note. FAST = Faculty of Applied Science and Textiles, FB = Faculty of Business, FCE = Faculty of Construction and Environment, FENG = Faculty of Engineering, FH = Faculty of Humanities, FHSS = Faculty of Health and Social Sciences, SD = School of Design, SHTM = School of Hotel and Tourism Management.

OUR STUDY

Participants were students enrolled in the four-year undergraduate curriculum at PolyU in the 2012-2013, 2013-2014, and 2014-2015 academic years. In the end of December 2014, a total of 480 students enrolled in the new four-year curriculum were randomly selected. 60 students were randomly selected from the student population of each of the eight faculties/schools from three cohorts, i.e., 2012-2013, 2013-2014, and 2014-2015 cohorts. These students were invited by phone and email to complete an online evaluation form. Up to the mid-January 2015, a total of 332 students completed the form. Due to the large amount of data and the different types of questions in the form, the present study was only based on students' responses to open-ended questions: "Do you have any memorable experiences in your study of GUR subjects? If 'yes,' would you share your experiences with us?" Among the 332 students who had completed the evaluation form, 240 students responded to the open-ended questions. The numbers of students responded to the questions by faculty and by cohort are listed in Table 1.

Instrument

The whole evaluation form was developed by the authors to collect students' views about different aspects of GUR implementation from both quantitative and qualitative approaches. Therefore, the form comprised both close-ended and open-ended questions. The close-ended questions focused on students' ratings of their understanding of the new four-year curriculum and the GUR. The open-ended questions focused on descriptors given by students to describe their impressions of the GUR and the open-ended questions on their memorable experiences in their study of GUR subjects. The present study focused on students' responses to the following open-ended questions: "Do you have any memorable experiences in your study of GUR subjects? If 'yes,' would you share your experiences with us?" This question was designed to understand the implementation and perceived effectiveness of the GUR from the perspective of the students.

Data analyses

All the responses were input into an Excel file. A postdoctoral fellow carefully read these responses for three times, and coded all responses into different themes. Responses under each theme were further coded into sub-themes. A more detailed description of each code was given below.

FINDINGS

Five themes emerged from the coding. They were "Active and Experiential Learning," "Interesting and Useful Contents," "Positive and Rich Learning

Outcomes," "Caring, Helpful and Qualified Teachers," and "Challenges." The following part elaborates these themes one by one.

Active and experiential learning

A majority of students expressed that they had gained most memorable experiences through joining different kinds of active and experiential learning activities in GUR. Firstly, students perceived that most of GUR subjects adopted group project works in their teaching and assessment sections. These group project experiences were "interesting" and helpful to students' competences in thinking and teamwork. This can be illustrated by the following responses:

- "Yes. Most of GUR subjects consist of group projects which I found interesting to work with others."
- "In CAR subject, we were given a whole tutorial session to present our findings and the classmates could discuss our findings and voice out different opinions. That was memorable."
- "Have a 'formal' project in FS and Tomorrow's Leaders which can experience the attitude and how to work together, so that I can have experience in doing project in the next few years."

Students also expressed that the experiential learning experiences, particularly those offered by Service Learning subjects, confronted them with people in different cultures and situations. Particularly, by helping underprivileged people in local and foreign cultures, students had most striking memorizations in learning. They did more self-reflection on their current life, learned contribution and appreciation, and developed sense of meaning and achievement. These perceptions of students are illustrated by the following responses:

- "In Service Learning, I met a good lecturer with [a] great course. I went to Sichuan and conducted service there. I learned so many things through the lectures and the service trip there. I had experienced something I won't forget, lifelong lasting and meaningful."

- "Service Learning is the most meaningful and valuable subject among all GUR subjects. I learn to appreciate and contribute. I think the school can put more emphasis on this subject."
- "Service Learning provides a great chance for me to live in village in Indonesia which was an unforgettable experience that I would never have in the future. It lets me reflect on myself that I have owned a lot in Hong Kong and treasure what I have now. Thanks for the SL subject."

Students were also impressed by other experiential learning activities, such as fieldwork. For example, two students consistently expressed that their most memorable experience in GUR study was coming from the fieldwork experience in one CAR subject named *First Bucket of Gold in China*. Through the fieldwork, the students experienced local culture in China and "understand the enterprises in Hangzhou." Students also enjoyed very much about some CAR subjects that combined experiential learning and high quality class-teaching. This is illustrated by the following narratives:

- "The subject *First Bucket of Gold in China* was really impressive. There was a trip to Hangzhou. The trip provided a lot of chances for us to understand the enterprises in Hangzhou and was very interesting. The workload was suitable and the lecturer could explain the theories very clearly. It is also very practical for our future."
- "The *Chinese Wisdom* is the course I enjoyed the most with a lively teaching and field trips."

Interesting and useful contents

Students generally had positive perceptions of the content of GUR subjects. They showed their fondness of subject contents in TL, HL, and CAR components. Students thought that the topics in TL subject were inspiring and reflective. The knowledge and skills learned from the subject could be applied to students' daily life, as shared in the following responses:

- "Among these subjects, *Tomorrow's Leaders* is my favorite subject as it is really useful in my daily life. In daily life, I have faced some emotional problem[s] which I could not deal with. However, during the lesson, I got help from this lesson. It helped me to find out the best way to solve the problem. This experience is really memorable and meaningful to me."
- "Yes, lectures of *Tomorrow's Leaders* are inspiring and help me reflect what is lacking in my intrapersonal development."

Students also expressed their fondness of HLS component, particularly for the sports-skills training session. Actually, to make the component more attractive, the HLS component was designed to have incorporated many novel and interesting sports skills in its sports-skills training session, such as Fencing, Frisbee, and Squash. Students gained great fun from doing and playing these sports skills. They also established a close relationship with their peers in the classes, as expressed in the following responses:

- "Yes, the sports skills class (fencing) is a very good experience. Fencing is an uncommon sport in secondary schools and I am really pleased that GUR offered such a course!"
- "Having squash classes at university made me feel like going back to the time in secondary school. I had great fun with other classmates and we laughed a lot during the sports skills training course."

Some students also perceived that the topics in some CAR subjects were interesting and exposed them to new area of knowledge, as shared in the following responses:

- "Attending *The Evolution of World Cuisine* is very great because I had chance to try many new things."

- "Cluster Area Requirements (CAR) course *Court and Palace: Power and Intrigue in Imperial China* gives me a valuable learning experience."
- "The course, *Introduction to Sociology APSS112*, is memorable, a whole new area of study."

Positive and rich learning outcomes

A set of positive learning outcomes from the GUR were identified from students' responses. These included broadened knowledge base and horizon, writing and speaking skills, teamwork skills, interpersonal relationship, healthy lifestyle, social responsibility and a changed attitude towards life. For example, some students responded that:

- "I think the study of GUR subjects is far different from the past. It is more diverse, so that I can broaden my horizons."
- "CAR-D course provides me a lot and it triggers me a new route in my life."
- "*Tomorrow's Leaders* helps build up inter- and intra-personal relationship."

Interestingly, it could be identified that there was a relationship between active and experiential learning activities and students' development of learning outcomes in their GUR study. For example, through Service Learning, particularly through experiencing different cultures and helping underprivileged people in service activities, a few students learned how to treasure their current life and developed sense of responsibility to the society. One student shared his response as follows:

- "In last semester, I joined a Service Learning course, [during] which [I] went to Qinghai and Guizhou to provide vision screening for local students. It was joyful and memorable experience for me because it was the first time I went to do voluntary work in China. I felt my work has greater purpose other than getting good grades and the joy from helping others is unforgettable."

Different group projects and writing assessments in different GUR subjects provided plenty of opportunities for students to practice their teamwork, writing skills and oral expression skills, as shared by following responses.

- "I wrote from the beginning to the end, total 12 pages in the final exam of a CAR subject, it is amazing!"
- "Yes, I have written a long story in creative writing course and I gained a high satisfaction."
- In the study of Freshman Seminar, once we were hoped to describe 'creativity.' It was the first time I stood in front of many people to speak out my innermost thoughts and feelings. This impressed me and encouraged me."
- "It is nice to cooperate with others in Freshman Seminar and it is very memorable to work with my groupmates overnight in order to finish our work and to have final adjustment."

Caring, helpful and qualified teachers

Students had very positive impression of some of their GUR teachers. They were deeply impressed by these teachers' caring and helpful attitude and appreciated it very much. This was illustrated by the following narratives:

- "Alice (alias for confidentiality) who is one of the instructors of *Tomorrow's Leaders* is very nice and helpful."
- "Except [for] one CAR teacher, all the other CAR teachers that have taught me were very passionate and helpful. They knew our needs and were eager to provide learning materials."

- "The most memorable experience in my GUR subject study is *Tomorrow's Leaders*, as the lecturer is nice and tries to invite us to share our story."

Some teachers' qualified teaching and caring attitudes also promoted students' deep and active learning of the subjects. This has been illustrated by the following responses:

- "I particularly enjoyed *Tomorrow's Leaders* subject, and my lecturer has been very motivating and sincere during lectures. I learned a lot about life and being a good leader and did a lot of meaningful reflections."
- "My English teacher, John (alias for confidentiality), is a very patient and caring teacher. His way of teaching makes the learning atmosphere very relaxing and good. He makes students communicate well with one another."
- "Yes, my lecturer in Freshman Seminar appreciated our efforts of deliberating a good presentation. And I really appreciated her for treating me, my teammates, and the free rider fairly."

Challenges

Two major challenges in studying GUR subjects emerged from the student responses. The first challenge was students' difficulty in subject registration of CAR subjects. Several students perceived that it was difficult for them to register the CAR subjects which they were interested in. Besides, difficulties in fulfilling the Reading and Writing Requirements and China Studies Requirements of CAR were noted. Serious timetable clashes between many CAR subjects and students' other prescribed subjects were also shown by the findings. Some students also encountered difficulties in registering HLS subjects. They worried whether they could fulfill the requirements of HLS on time as shared in the following responses:

- "I couldn't register Healthy Lifestyle [courses] in every semester. All the vacancies were taken by people. Please open more vacancies. And I always get time crash with the pre-assigned subjects and the CAR and Service Learning subjects. It is hard to prepare a good timetable."
- "Hard to register the CAR subject I want and fulfill the requirement. Always zero vacancy."

Another challenge mentioned by some of the students was the reluctant or negative attitudes towards studying GUR subjects, particularly when the CAR subjects were far beyond their own majors. Particularly, a few students majoring in social sciences or humanities expressed their unwillingness of studying science subjects in CAR-D area. They had less interest in studying science subjects because they could not perceive the relationship between these subjects and their majors and they had a weak background on science. This can be illustrated by a response below:

- "In fact I am an APSS student and I find it useless for us to study CAR-D [subjects]. We should not be asked to learn CAR-D right? It's a trap for those who are interested in social science as a number of us are bad at science."

Discussion

The present study investigated how students perceived the General University Requirements (GUR) in the new four-year undergraduate curriculum at The Hong Kong Polytechnic University (PolyU). Several major observations were gained from the findings. Primarily, students perceived that active and experiential teaching and learning methods widely adopted in GUR subjects (such as group project work and service learning) were very useful. These methods facilitated student learning in the GUR. They also promoted students' development in a variety of inter- and intra-personal competences such as thinking, teamwork, civic value, and self-reflection. This finding was in line with other qualitative findings on GUR in the same and different years (21-23).

The findings have two implications. First, the findings indicated that GUR at PolyU was generally effective in promoting students' inter- and intra-personal development. Second, the findings suggested that active and experiential teaching and learning methods were a key factor to effectiveness of general education courses. The findings are in line with the general scientific literature. For example, research suggests that Service Learning had positive impacts on a variety of aspects of student development including social competence, social responsibility, ability to work with students with diversified backgrounds, cognitive complexity, self-assurance and personal efficacy (24-26). Results from the present study further strengthened these findings by showing that Service Learning experiences changed students' attitudes towards life, promoted their self-reflections on life and society, and helped them break through their own narrowness to concern more about the society and others.

Secondly, students had positive perceptions about the subject contents of the GUR. Particularly, they perceived the contents of some GUR subjects, such as Tomorrow's Leaders (TL), as much useful and applicable to their daily life. The subject helped students reflect on their intra- and inter-personal development and helped them tackle their developmental problems. Research found that the emotional and anxiety problems of first-year undergraduate students in Hong Kong were relatively high (27). Based on the positive youth development approach, the rationale of TL subject was to promote students' leadership and intrapersonal competences. Existing studies suggested that TL subject was positively evaluated by students in terms of its learning experiences and achievement of intended learning outcomes (28, 29). Previous studies also showed that TL subject was effective in promoting students' inter- and intra-personal development, self-reflection and self-understanding (30, 31). Findings from the present study further strengthened these existing findings by showing how students benefited from TL subject based on qualitative research findings.

Thirdly, teacher was another important factor to the effectiveness of the GUR. Findings of the present study suggested that caring attitude and behavior of some teachers greatly facilitated students' learning and personal development. This observation is consistent with the literature suggesting that teachers' caring behavior was influential to students' development. For example, research indicates that caring teachers could strengthen teacher-student relationships, increase students' confidence in teachers, and increase students' motivation to succeed (32). Studies also found that teachers showing more enthusiasm about teaching would deliver higher quality of teaching (33) and foster more meaningful learning of students (34). Enthusiastic teachers provide stimulus that attracts the attention of students, and promotes students' adaptation as well as experience of their enthusiastic attitudes and emotions, which would facilitate students' deep engagement in learning (33).

Finally, two major challenges were identified in the implementation of the GUR. One challenge was students' registration of CAR and HLS subjects. This might be due to several possible reasons. Firstly, students' subject registration in CAR was restricted by the "multiple" requirements. For example, although there were many CAR subjects on offer in each academic year, only about one third of these subjects had English reading and writing requirements, and less than one third of these subjects had Chinese reading and writing requirements. In order to fulfill the multiple requirements of CAR, students had to select from the subjects with English and Chinese reading and writing requirements. This limited the scope of their selection. Secondly, students' tight study schedule in one semester was also a reason for their difficulty in registering CAR subjects. Although there were many CAR subjects on offer, students had to choose those that fit into their busy schedule. Meanwhile, these subjects should also fulfill reading and writing requirements. This increased students' difficulty in registering CAR subjects. The other challenge was a few students' negative attitudes towards studying science subjects in CAR because they majored in humanities and social sciences. One reason might be that some science subjects in CAR were designed with a more advanced content which was far beyond social science students' knowledge background. Although it is a challenge to deliver science subject to non-science major students, careful revision on science subjects and related faculty training should be conducted to promote students' learning in this area. Despite these challenges, findings of the present study suggest that the implementation of the GUR is smooth and effective from students' perspective.

Acknowledgments

The authors thank The Hong Kong Polytechnic University for providing financial support via the Teaching Development Grant in conducting the longitudinal GUR evaluation study. The materials in this chapter are based on a paper published in the *International Journal on Disability and Human Development* 2017;16 (4) issue.

References

[1] Wehlburg CM. Integrated general education: A brief look back. New Dir Teach Learn 2010;121:3-11.

[2] Harvard Committee. General education in a free society: Report of the Harvard Committee. Cambridge, MA: Harvard University Press, 1946.

[3] Hutchins RM. The higher learning in America. J High Educ 1999;70(5):524-32.

[4] Stevens AH. The philosophy of general education and its contradictions: The influence of Hutchins. J Gen Educ 2001;50:165-91.

[5] Boyer EL, Levine A. A quest for common learning. Change: Mag High Learn 1981;13(3):28-35.

[6] McGrath EJ. The general education movement (An editorial). J Gen Educ 1946;1:3-8.

[7] Newton RR. Tensions and models in general education planning. J Gen Educ 2000;49:165-81.

[8] Brubacher JS. On the philosophy of higher education, revised Ed. San Francisco, CA: Jossey-Bass, 1982.

[9] Xing J, Ng P, Cheng C (Eds). General education and the development of global citizenship in Hong Kong, Taiwan and mainland China: Not merely icing on the cake. London: Routledge, 2013.

[10] Association of American Colleges and Universities. College learning for the new global century: A report from the National Leadership Council for Liberal Education

and America's Promise, 2007. URL: https://www.aacu.org/sites/default/files/files/LEAP/GlobalCentury_final.pdf.

[11] Jaffee D. The general education initiative in Hong Kong: Organized contradictions and emerging tensions. High Educ 2012;64:193-206.

[12] Twombly SB. General education: The insiders' view. New Dir High Educ 1992;80:91-103.

[13] Twombly SB. Student perspectives on general education in a research university: An exploratory study. J Gen Educ 1992;41:238-72.

[14] King LO, Kotrlik JW. Relevance of the general education core curriculum to career goals of college of agriculture students. J Agr Educ 1995;36:26-33.

[15] Vander Schee BA. Changing general education perceptions through "perspectives" and the interdisciplinary first-year seminar. Int J Teach Learn High Educ 2011;23:382-7.

[16] Astin AW, Vogelgesang LJ, Ikeda EK, Yee JA. How service learning affects students. University of Nebraska Omaha, 2000. URL: http://digitalcommons.unomaha.edu/cgi/viewcontent.cgi?article=1145&context=slcehighered.

[17] Moely BE, McFarland M, Miron D, Mercer S, Ilustre V. Changes in college students' attitudes and intentions for civic involvement as a function of service-learning experiences. Mich J Commun Serv Learn 2002;9:18-26.

[18] Shek DTL, Yu L. General university requirements and holistic development in university students in Hong Kong. Int J Adolesc Med Health 2017;29(1):41-8. DOI: 10.1515/ijamh-2017-3006.

[19] Shek DTL, Yu L. The impact of 3-year and 4-year undergraduate programs on university students: The case of Hong Kong. Int J Adolesc Med Health 2017; 29(1):49-55. DOI: 10.1515/ijamh-2017-3007.

[20] Shek DTL, Yu L, Ngai J. Evaluation of a general education program in Hong Kong: Secondary data analyses based on student feedback questionnaires. Int J Disabil Hum Dev 2015;14:401-6.

[21] Shek DTL, Yu L, Chai WY. Evaluation of the general university requirements: What did students say? Int J Adolesc Med Health 2017;29(1):75-82. DOI: 10.1515/ijamh-2017-3010.

[22] Shek DTL, Yu L, Wu FKY, Chai WY. General University Requirements at The Hong Kong Polytechnic University: Evaluation findings based on student focus groups. Assess Eval High Educ 2015;40:1017-31.

[23] Shek DTL, Lu Y, Zhu X. Qualitative evaluation of a new general education program in Hong Kong: Findings based on students. Int J Child Adolesc Health 2017;10(3):347-56.

[24] Eyler J, Giles DE, Stenson CM, Gray CJ. At a glance: What we know about the effects of service-learning on college students, faculty, institutions and communities, 1993-2000: Third edition. University of Nebraska Omaha, 2001. URL: http://digitalcommons.unomaha.edu/cgi/viewcontent.cgi?article=1137&context=slcehighered

[25] Kendrick JRJr. Outcomes of service-learning in an introduction to sociology course. Mich J Commun Serv Learn 1996;3:72-81.

[26] Osborne RE, Hammerich S, Hensley C. Student effects of service-learning: Tracking change across a semester. Mich J Commun Serv Learn 1998;5:5-13.

[27] Shek DTL, Sun RCF, Chui YH, Lit SW, Yuen WW, Chung YYH, et al. Development and evaluation of a positive youth development course for university students in Hong Kong. ScientificWorldJournal 2012;8. DOI: 10.1100/2012/263731.

[28] Shek DTL, Yu L. Student feedback on a subject on leadership and intrapersonal development for university students in Hong Kong. Int J Disabil Hum Dev 2016;15:339-46.

[29] Shek DTL, Yu L, Xie QZ. Student feedback on a pioneer subject on leadership and intrapersonal development in Hong Kong. Int J Adolesc Med Health 2017;29(1):83-9. DOI: 10.1515/ijamh-2017-3011.

[30] Shek DTL, Sun RCF. Focus group evaluation of a positive youth development course in a university in Hong Kong. Int J Disabil Hum Dev 2012;11:249-54.

[31] Shek DTL, Sun RCF. Promoting psychological competencies in university students: Evaluation based on a one-group pre-test/post-test design. Int J Disabil Hum Dev 2012;11:229-34.

[32] Owens LM, Ennis CD. The ethic of care in teaching: An overview of supportive literature. Quest 2005;57:392-425.

[33] Kunter M, Tsai, YM, Klusmann U, Brunner M, Krauss S, Baumert J. Students' and mathematics teachers' perceptions of teacher enthusiasm and instruction. Learn Instr 2008;18:468-82.

[34] Keller M, Neumann K, Fischer HE. Teacher enthusiasm and student learning. In: Hattie J, Anderman EM, eds. International guide to student achievement. New York: Routledge, 2013:247-9.

SECTION FIVE: ACKNOWLEDGMENTS

In: Soft Skills and Aspirations … ISBN: 978-1-53614-092-7
Editors: Daniel TL Shek, et al.

Chapter 14

ABOUT THE EDITORS

Daniel TL Shek, PhD, FHKPS, BBS, SBS, JP, is Associate Vice President (undergraduate Programme), Chair Professor of Applied Social Sciences, and Li and Fung Professor in Service Leadership Education, the Hong Kong Polytechnic University, Hunghom, Hong Kong, PRC, Advisory Professor of East China Normal University, Honorary Professor of Kiang Wu Nursing College of Macau and Adjunct Professor, Division of Adolescent Medicine, Department of Pediatrics, University of Kentucky College of Medicine, Lexington, United States. He is Chief Editor of *Journal of Youth Studies* and *Applied Research in Quality of Life*, past Consulting Editor of *Journal of Clinical Psychology*, and editorial board member of *Social Indicators Research, International Journal of Adolescent Medicine and Health, Asian Journal of Counseling, International Journal of Disability and Human Development,* and *International Journal of Adolescent Medicine and Health*. He has served in many government advisory bodies, including the Action Committee against Narcotics, Commission on Youth, Fight Crime Committee and Family Council. He has published numerous books, book chapters and more than 500 scientific articles in international refereed journals. Email: daniel.shek@polyu.edu.hk

Janet TY Leung, PhD, RSW, is the Associate Professor of the Department of Applied Social Sciences in The Hong Kong Polytechnic University. She obtained her PhD in social work from The Hong Kong Polytechnic University. She is a registered social worker and was a service supervisor in a social service organization, responsible for service planning and supervising a wide range of services such as children and youth services, school counseling services, training projects for dyslexic children, family support programmes, service for the homeless people, community development projects etc. Her areas of interest include poverty, adolescent development, family processes and parent education. Her work appears in *Research on Social Work Practice, British Journal of Social Work, Journal of Youth and Adolescence, Journal of Family Issues, and Journal of Child and Family Studies*. Email: janet.leung@polyu.edu.hk

Joav Merrick, MD, MMedSci, DMSc, born and educated in Denmark is professor of pediatrics, Division of Pediatrics, Hadassah Hebrew University Medical Center, Mt Scopus Campus, Jerusalem, Israel and Kentucky Children's Hospital, University of Kentucky, Lexington, Kentucky, United States and professor of public health at the Center for Healthy Development, School of Public Health, Georgia State University, Atlanta, United States, the former medical director of the Health Services, Division for Intellectual and Developmental Disabilities, Ministry of Social Affairs and Social Services, Jerusalem, the founder and director of the National Institute of Child Health and Human Development in Israel. Numerous publications in the field of pediatrics, child health and human development, rehabilitation, intellectual disability, disability, health, welfare, abuse, advocacy, quality of life and prevention. Received the Peter Sabroe Child Award for outstanding work on behalf of Danish Children in 1985 and the International LEGO-Prize ("The Children's Nobel Prize") for an extraordinary contribution towards improvement in child welfare and well-being in 1987. In 2017 appointed a Kentucky Colonel by the Commonwealth of Kentucky, the highest honor the governor can bestow to a person. Email: jmerrick@zahav.net.il

In: Soft Skills and Aspirations … ISBN: 978-1-53614-092-7
Editors: Daniel TL Shek, et al.

Chapter 15

About the Department of Applied Social Sciences, The Hong Kong Polytechnic University, Hunghom, Hong Kong

The Department of Applied Social Sciences (APSS) of the Hong Kong Polytechnic University began as the Institute of Social Work Training in 1973 before it became the School of Social Work in the Hong Kong Polytechnic in 1977. In 1986, the department was renamed as the Department of Applied Social Sciences. It is now one of the largest social science departments in the Asia-Pacific region with a strong tradition of researching on and working with socially vulnerable groups through education, research and service in diverse areas incorporating social work, social policy and administration, psychology, sociology and philosophy.

Education

In education, we strive to nurture human service professionals who are knowledgeable, resourceful, caring, worldly but reflexive, and possess a strong commitment to social justice and responsibility. We also see them as practitioners and researchers who are able to integrate theory and practice, and develop appropriate indigenous knowledge that can meet the challenges of rapid social change in Chinese societies.

Research

In research, to respond to the constantly changing global socio-economic order and addressing the subsequently emerged local problems, the strategic foci of our research and social investigation have also been expanded to include migration and mobilities, family and life-span development, social economy, online communities/social media, disaster and risks reduction, applied philosophy and social work practices.

Community Service

In community service, we continue to collaborate with community partners to allow our students to understand better the different worlds of our society, design programmes and supportive services that are innovative, relevant and socially responsible.

Students

As students in our department, we see it necessary for them to develop a global outlook while firmly grounded in Hong Kong. To this end, in recent years more than 200 full-time and part-time students as well as alumni have participated in the various study tours and exchange programmes we held in the Chinese Mainland and overseas, including the University of Nottingham, United Kingdom; University of Queensland, Australia; University of California at Berkeley, United States; Washington University at St. Louis,

United States; York University, Canada; Peking University and Yunnan University in China.

FACULTY AND TEACHING

In the 2017/18 academic year, the Department has more than 200 members, including academic staff, part-time fieldwork instructors, research and project staff and administrative and supporting technical staff. The APSS offers undergraduate, and coursework-based or research-based post-graduate. Over the years, more than 14,000 students have graduated.

In: Soft Skills and Aspirations … ISBN: 978-1-53614-092-7
Editors: Daniel TL Shek, et al.

Chapter 16

ABOUT THE NATIONAL INSTITUTE OF CHILD HEALTH AND HUMAN DEVELOPMENT IN ISRAEL

The National Institute of Child Health and Human Development (NICHD) in Israel was established in 1998 as a virtual institute under the auspices of the Medical Director, Ministry of Social Affairs and Social Services in order to function as the research arm for the Office of the Medical Director. In 1998 the National Council for Child Health and Pediatrics, Ministry of Health and in 1999 the Director General and Deputy Director General of the Ministry of Health endorsed the establishment of the NICHD.

MISSION

The mission of a National Institute for Child Health and Human Development in Israel is to provide an academic focal point for the scholarly interdisciplinary study of child life, health, public health, welfare, disability, rehabilitation, intellectual disability and related aspects of human development. This mission includes research, teaching, clinical work, information and public service activities in the field of child health and human development.

SERVICE AND ACADEMIC ACTIVITIES

Over the years many activities became focused in the south of Israel due to collaboration with various professionals at the Faculty of Health Sciences (FOHS) at the Ben Gurion University of the Negev (BGU). Since 2000 an affiliation with the Zusman Child Development Center at the Pediatric Division of Soroka University Medical Center has resulted in collaboration around the establishment of the Down Syndrome Clinic at that center. In 2002 a full course on "Disability" was established at the Recanati School for Allied Professions in the Community, FOHS, BGU and in 2005 collaboration was started with the Primary Care Unit of the faculty and disability became part of the master of public health course on "Children and society". In the academic year 2005-2006 a one semester course on "Aging with disability" was started as part of the master of science program in gerontology in our collaboration with the Center for Multidisciplinary Research in Aging. In 2010 collaborations with the Division of Pediatrics, Hadassah Hebrew University Medical Center, Jerusalem, Israel around the National Down Syndrome Center and taught students and residents about intellectual and developmental disabilities as part of their training at this campus.

RESEARCH ACTIVITIES

The affiliated staff have over the years published work from projects and research activities in this national and international collaboration. In the year 2000 the *International Journal of Adolescent Medicine and Health* and in 2005 the *International Journal on Disability and Human Development* of De Gruyter Publishing House (Berlin and New York) were affiliated with the National Institute of Child Health and Human Development. From 2008 also the *International Journal of Child Health and Human Development* (Nova Science Publishers, Inc., New York), the *International Journal of Child and Adolescent Health* (Nova Science Publishers, Inc.) and the *Journal of Pain Management* (Nova Science Publishers, Inc.) and from 2009 the *International Public Health Journal* (Nova Science Publishers, Inc.) and *Journal of Alternative Medicine Research* (Nova Science Publishers, Inc.) were affiliated. All are peer-reviewed international journals.

NATIONAL COLLABORATIONS

Nationally the NICHD works in collaboration with the Faculty of Health Sciences, Ben Gurion University of the Negev; Department of Physical Therapy, Sackler School of Medicine, Tel Aviv University; Autism Center, Assaf HaRofeh Medical Center; National Rett and PKU Centers at Chaim Sheba Medical Center, Tel HaShomer; Department of Physiotherapy, Haifa University; Department of Education, Faculty of Social Sciences and Health Sciences, Bar Ilan University, Ramat Gan; College of Judea and Samaria in Ariel and in 2011 affiliation with Center for Pediatric Chronic Diseases and National Center for Down Syndrome, Department of Pediatrics, Hadassah Hebrew University Medical Center, Mount Scopus Campus, Jerusalem.

INTERNATIONAL COLLABORATIONS

Internationally with the Department of Disability and Human Development, College of Applied Health Sciences, University of Illinois at Chicago; Strong Center for Developmental Disabilities, Golisano Children's Hospital at Strong, University of Rochester School of Medicine and Dentistry, New York; Centre on Intellectual Disabilities, University of Albany, New York; Centre for Chronic Disease Prevention and Control, Health Canada, Ottawa; Chandler Medical Center and Children's Hospital, Kentucky Children's

Hospital, Section of Adolescent Medicine, University of Kentucky, Lexington; Chronic Disease Prevention and Control Research Center, Baylor College of Medicine, Houston, Texas; Division of Neuroscience, Department of Psychiatry, Columbia University, New York; Institute for the Study of Disadvantage and Disability, Atlanta; Center for Autism and Related Disorders, Department Psychiatry, Children's Hospital Boston, Boston; Department of Pediatric and Adolescent Medicine, Western Michigan University Homer Stryker MD School of Medicine, Kalamazoo, Michigan, United States; Department of Paediatrics, Child Health and Adolescent Medicine, Children's Hospital at Westmead, Westmead, Australia; International Centre for the Study of Occupational and Mental Health, Düsseldorf, Germany; Centre for Advanced Studies in Nursing, Department of General Practice and Primary Care, University of Aberdeen, Aberdeen, United Kingdom; Quality of Life Research Center, Copenhagen, Denmark; Nordic School of Public Health, Gottenburg, Sweden, Scandinavian Institute of Quality of Working Life, Oslo, Norway; The Department of Applied Social Sciences (APSS) of the Hong Kong Polytechnic University, Hong Kong.

Targets

Our focus is on research, international collaborations, clinical work, teaching and policy in health, disability and human development and to establish the NICHD as a permanent institute in Israel in order to conduct model research and policy.

Contact

Professor Joav Merrick, MD, MMedSci, DMSc
Director, National Institute of Child Health and Human Development, Jerusalem, Israel.
Email: jmerrick@zahav.net.il

In: Soft Skills and Aspirations … ISBN: 978-1-53614-092-7
Editors: Daniel TL Shek, et al.

Chapter 17

About the Book Series "Pediatrics, Child and Adolescent Health"

Pediatrics, child and adolescent health is a book series with publications from a multidisciplinary group of researchers, practitioners and clinicians for an international professional forum interested in the broad spectrum of pediatric medicine, child health, adolescent health and human development.

- Merrick J, ed. *Child and adolescent health yearbook 2011.* New York: Nova Science Publishers, Inc., 2012.
- Merrick J, ed. *Child and adolescent health yearbook 2012.* New York: Nova Science Publishers, Inc., 2012.
- Roach RR, Greydanus DE, Patel DR, Homnick DN, Merrick J, eds. *Tropical pediatrics: A public health concern of international proportions.* New York: Nova Science Publishers, Inc., 2012.
- Merrick J, ed. *Child health and human development yearbook 2011.* New York: Nova Science Publishers, Inc., 2012.
- Merrick J, ed. *Child health and human development yearbook 2012.* New York: Nova Science Publishers, Inc., 2012.

- Shek DTL, Sun RCF, Merrick J, eds. *Developmental issues in Chinese adolescents.* New York: Nova Science Publishers, Inc., 2012.
- Shek DTL, Sun RCF, Merrick J, eds. *Positive youth development: Theory, research and application.* New York: Nova Science Publishers, Inc., 2012.
- Zachor DA, Merrick J, eds. *Understanding autism spectrum disorder: Current research aspects*. New York: Nova Science Publishers, Inc., 2012.
- Ma HK, Shek DTL, Merrick J, eds. *Positive youth development: A new school curriculum to tackle adolescent developmental issues.* New York: Nova Science Publishers, Inc., 2012.
- Wood D, Reiss JG, Ferris ME, Edwards LR, Merrick J, eds. *Transition from pediatric to adult medical care.* New York: Nova Science Publishers, Inc., 2012.
- Isenberg Y. *Guidelines for the healthy integration of the ill child in the educational system: Experience from Israel*. New York: Nova Science Publishers, Inc., 2013.
- Shek DTL, Sun RCF, Merrick J, eds. *Chinese adolescent development: Economic disadvantages, parents and intrapersonal development.* New York: Nova Science Publishers, Inc., 2013.
- Shek DTL, Sun RCF, Merrick J, eds. *University and college students: Health and development issues for the leaders of tomorrow.* New York: Nova Science Publishers, Inc., 2013.
- Shek DTL, Sun RCF, Merrick J, eds. *Adolescence and behavior issues in a Chinese context.* New York: Nova Science Publishers, Inc., 2013.
- Sun J, Buys N, Merrick J. *Advances in preterm infant research*. New York: Nova Science Publishers, Inc., 2013.
- Tsitsika A, Janikian M, Greydanus DE, Omar HA, Merrick J, eds. *Internet addiction: A public health concern in adolescence*. New York: Nova Science Publishers, Inc., 2013.

- Shek DTL, Lee TY, Merrick J, eds. *Promotion of holistic development of young people in Hong Kong*. New York: Nova Science Publishers, Inc., 2013.
- Shek DTL, Ma C, Lu Y, Merrick J, eds. *Human developmental research: Experience from research in Hong Kong*. New York: Nova Science Publishers, Inc., 2013.
- Rubin IL, Merrick J, eds. *Child health and human development: Social, economic and environmental factors*. New York: Nova Science Publishers, Inc., 2013.
- Merrick J, ed. *Chronic disease and disability in childhood.* New York: Nova Science Publishers, Inc., 2013.
- Rubin IL, Merrick J, eds. *Break the cycle of environmental health disparities: Maternal and child health aspects*. New York: Nova Science Publishers, Inc., 2013.
- Rubin IL, Merrick J, eds. *Environmental health disparities in children: Asthma, obesity and food.* New York: Nova Science Publishers, Inc., 2013.
- Rubin IL, Merrick J, eds. *Environmental health: Home, school and community*. New York: Nova Science Publishers, Inc., 2013.
- Merrick J, Kandel I, Omar HA, eds. *Children, violence and bullying: International perspectives.* New York: Nova Science Publishers, Inc., 2013.
- Omar HA, Bowling CH, Merrick J, eds. *Playing with fire: Children, adolescents and firesetting.* New York: Nova Science Publishers, Inc., 2013.
- Merrick J, Tenenbaum A, Omar HA, eds. *School, adolescence and health issues.* New York: Nova Science Publishers, Inc., 2014.
- Merrick J, Tenenbaum A, Omar HA, eds. *Adolescence and sexuality: International perspectives.* New York: Nova Science Publishers, Inc., 2014.
- Diamond G, Arbel E. *Adoption: The search for a new parenthood adoption.* New York: Nova Science Publishers, Inc., 2014.

- Taylor MF, Pooley JA, Merrick J, eds. *Adolescence: Places and spaces*. New York: Nova Science Publishers, Inc., 2014.
- Greydanus DE, Feinberg AN, Merrick J, eds. *Born into this world: Health issues*. New York: Nova Science Publishers, Inc., 2014.
- Greydanus DE, Feinberg AN, Merrick J, eds. *Caring for the newborn: A comprehensive guide for the clinician*. New York: Nova Science Publishers, Inc., 2014.
- Rubin IL, Merrick J, eds. *Environment and hope: Improving health, reducing AIDS and promoting food security in the world*. New York: Nova Science Publishers, Inc., 2014.
- Greydanus DE, Feinberg AN, Merrick J, eds. *Pediatric and adolescent dermatology: Some current issues*. New York: Nova Science Publishers, Inc., 2014.
- Roach RR, Greydanus DE, Patel DR, Merrick J, eds. *Tropical pediatrics: A public helath concern of international proportions*, 2nd edition. New York: Nova Science Publishers, Inc., 2015.
- Merrick J, ed. *Child and adolescent health issues: A tribute to the pediatrician Donald E Greydanus*. New York: Nova Science Publishers, Inc., 2015.
- Feinberg AN. *A pediatric resident pocket guide: Making the most of morning reports*. New York: Nova Science Publishers, Inc., 2015.
- Greydanus DE, Patel DR, Pratt HD, Calles Jr JL, Nazeer A, Merrick J, eds. *Behavioral pediatrics*, 4th edition. New York: Nova Science Publishers, Inc., 2015.
- Merrick J, ed. *Disability, chronic disease and human development*. New York: Nova Science Publishers, Inc., 2015.
- Hegamin-Younger C, Merrick J, eds.*Caribbean adolescents: Some public health concerns*. New York: Nova Science Publishers, Inc., 2015.
- Merrick J, ed. *Adolescence and health: Some international perspectives*. New York: Nova Science Publishers, Inc., 2015.
- Omar HA. *Youth suicide prevention: Everybody's business*. New York: Nova Science Publishers, Inc., 2015.

- Greydanus DE, Raj VMS, Merrick J, eds. *Chronic disease and disability: The pediatric kidney.* New York: Nova Science Publishers, Inc., 2015.
- Merrick J, ed. *Children and childhood: Some international aspects.* New York: Nova Science Publishers, Inc., 2016.
- Shek DTL, Lee TY, Merrick J, eds. *Children and adolescents: Future challenges.* New York: Nova Science Publishers, Inc., 2016.
- Shek DTL, Wu FKU, Leung JTY, Merrick J, eds. *Adolescence: Positive youth development programs in Chinese communities.* New York: Nova Science Publishers, Inc., 2016.
- Merrick J, Greydanus DE, eds. *Sexuality: Some international aspects.* New York: Nova Science Publishers, Inc., 2016.
- Harel-Fisch Y, Abdeen Z, Navot M. *Growing up in the Middle East: The daily lives and well-being of Israeli and Palestinian youth.* New York: Nova Science Publishers, Inc., 2016.
- Greydanus DE, Malhotra D, Merrick J, eds. *Chronic disease and disability: The pediatric heart.* New York: Nova Science Publishers, Inc., 2016.
- Greydanus DE, Kamboj MK, Merrick J, eds. *Chronic disease and disability: The pediatric pancreas.* New York: Nova Science Publishers, Inc., 2016.
- Kamboj MK, Greydanus DE, Merrick J, eds. *Diabetes mellitus: Childhood and adolescence.* New York: Nova Science Publishers, Inc., 2016.
- Greydanus DE, Palusci VJ, Merrick J, eds. *Chronic disease and disability: Abuse and neglect in childhood and adolescence.* New York: Nova Science Publishers, Inc., 2016.
- Greydanus DE, Calles JL Jr, Patel DR, Nazeer A, Merrick J, eds. *Clinical aspects of psychopharmacology in childhood and adolescence*, 2nd ed. New York: Nova Science Publishers, Inc., 2016.

- Greydanus DE, Apple RW, White K, Merrick J, eds. *Children and youth: Post-traumatic stress disorder and motor vehicle crashes.* New York: Nova Science Publishers, Inc., 2017.
- Mazaba ML, Siziya S, Merrick J, eds. *Suicide: A global view on suicidal ideation among adolescents.* New York: Nova Science Publishers, Inc., 2017.
- Chow R, Merrick J, eds. *Adolescence: Bicycle and helmet use of adolescents and young adults.* New York: Nova Science Publishers, Inc., 2017.
- Chow R, Borean M, Hollenberg D, Viehweger J, Anpalagan T, Rzepka A, Merrick J, eds. *Bicycles: Helmet use and adolescents at independent schools.* New York: Nova Science Publishers, Inc., 2017.
- Shek DTL, Ma CMS, Leung JTY, Merrick J, eds. *Positive youth development: Long term effects in a Chinese program.* New York: Nova Science Publishers, Inc., 2017.
- Greydanus DE, Atay O, Merrick J, eds. *Chronic disease and disability: The pediatric gastrointestinal tract.* New York: Nova Science Publishers, Inc., 2018.
- Omar HA, Chalkley J, eds. *Multiple sclerosis in children and adolescents.* New York: Nova Science Publishers, Inc., 2018.
- Merrick J, ed. *Childhood and adolescence: Tribute to Emanuel Chigier, 1928-2017.* New York: Nova Science Publishers, Inc., 2018.
- Greydanus DE, Gregoire-Bottex MM, Cates KW, Merrick J, eds. *Chronic disease and disability: The pediatric lung.* New York: Nova Science Publishers, Inc., 2018.
- Omar HA, Merrick J, eds. *Building youth for the future: A path towards suicide prevention.* New York: Nova Science Publishers, Inc., 2018.

CONTACT

Professor Joav Merrick, MD, MMedSci, DMSc
Director, National Institute of Child Health and Human Development, Jerusalem, Israel
Email: jmerrick@zahav.net.il

SECTION SIX: INDEX

INDEX

#

A

B

C

D

E

F

G

H

I

J

K

L

M

N

O

P

T

U

V

W

Y

Positive Youth Development: Long Term Effects in a Chinese Program

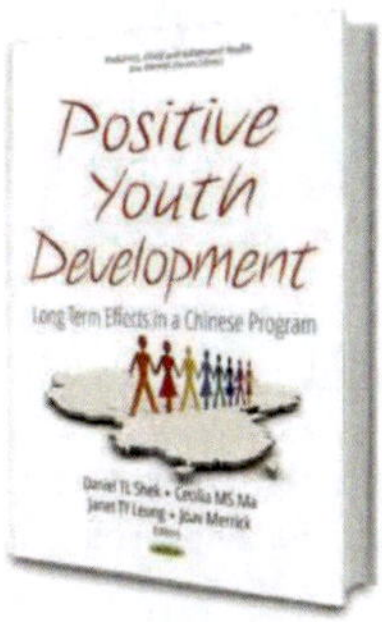

Editors: Daniel TL Shek, Ph.D., Cecilia MS Ma, Ph.D., Janet TY Leung, Ph.D., and Joav Merrick, M.D. (Medical Director, Health Services, Division for Intellectual and Developmental

Series: Pediatrics, Child and Adolescent Health

Book Description: In this book, the authors present the first known scientific study on the psychosocial development in Chinese adolescents in Hong Kong. A large sample was used and validated measures of positive youth development, family functioning, parent-child relational processes and adolescent risk behavior were included in the study.

Hardcover ISBN: 978-1-53612-539-9
Retail Price: $230

Adolescence: Positive Youth Development Programs in Chinese Communities

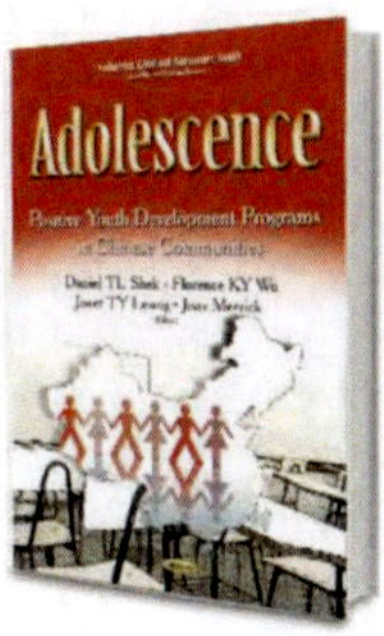

Editors: Daniel TL Shek, Florence KY Wu, Janet TY Leung, and Joav Merrick (Department of Applied Social Sciences, The Hong Kong Polytechnic University, Hong Kong, PR China, and others)

Series: Pediatrics, Child and Adolescent Health

Book Description: In this book, we present the training program in mainland China and also a leadership project for university students at The Hong Kong Polytechnic University. The chapters underscore the importance of evaluation, and we hope that the findings will motivate university teachers and others to utilize positive youth development principles within and outside of Hong Kong.

Hardcover ISBN: 978-1-63484-044-6
Retail Price: $190

Chinese Adolescent Development: Economic Disadvantages, Parents and Intrapersonal Development

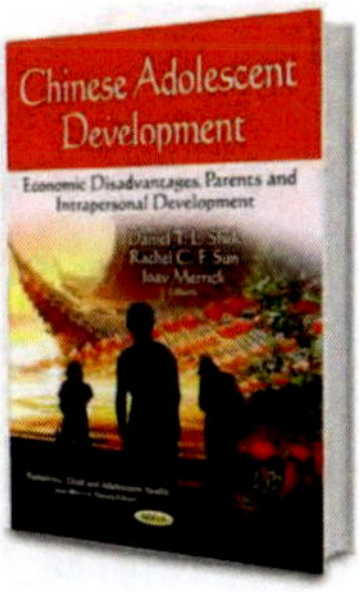

Editors: Daniel T.L. Shek, Rachel C.F. Sun and Joav Merrick (Health Services, Division for Intellectual and Developmental Disabilities, Ministry of Social Affairs and Social Services, Jerusalem, Israel, and others)

Series: Pediatrics, Child and Adolescent Health

Book Description: In this book, several papers reporting evaluation findings for the second piloting exercise are included. Because there are few validated positive youth development programs in the Chinese context, it is our modest wish that the accumulated evidence can give us some insights about the usefulness of having positive youth development subjects designed for university students.

Hardcover ISBN: 978-1-62618-622-4
Retail Price: $179

Adolescence and Behavior Issues in a Chinese Context

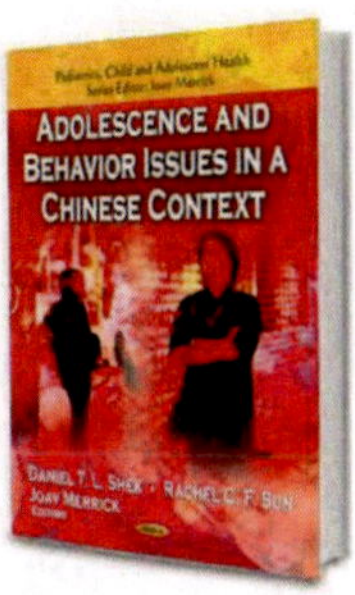

Editors: Daniel T.L. Shek, Rachel C.F. Sun, and Joav Merrick (Health Services, Division for Intellectual and Developmental Disabilities, Ministry of Social Affairs and Social Services, Jerusalem, Israel, and others)

Series: Pediatrics, Child and Adolescent Health

Book Description: Adopting the ecological approach, adolescents' behaviors result from the complex interplay between themselves and the surrounding environment. These issues will be addressed in this book with experience from research from Hong Kong in a Chinese context.

Hardcover ISBN: 978-1-62618-614-9
Retail Price: $205